# My Health and Fitness

## Volume 3

### 53 Articles

## By: Wade Yoder

### Master Trainer - Fitness Nutrition Specialist

### - Health & Fitness Columnist

**Dedicated to:** the discouraged, the scared, the financially strapped, the hurting, the confused, the frustrated and last but not least, the ones who feel that spending a major amount of their life in doctor's office waiting rooms and endless diagnosis's is the new norm...

This book and series is dedicated to helping everyone I can to realize the power of the body's own resources when given the simple basics that it craves, such as the body's capability to fight premature aging and chronic disease, by formulating its own drugs through the power of the immune system.

Health, fitness, muscle building and weight loss should not be looked at as something that costs a lot of money. Our health and fitness is adaptive to the habits we adopt.

If this book helps make your path to health and fitness an easier less complicated one, then my mission is accomplished~ Wade Yoder

# Table of Contents

# Basic Year Round Health and Fitness Tips

**1. Immune system:** our immune system builds its intelligence by exposure to our surroundings. It becomes weak like an unused muscle when it remains unexposed. A completely sanitized environment is to the immune system like a gym (that has no equipment) is to our muscle. Diet, exposure and rest all work together to keep our immune system strong!

**2. Our back and neck:** our back and neck should be looked at as one of our most guarded investments, since it is through these that the brain sends its messages whether voluntary or involuntary for almost all of our life functions. Learning and using the plank properly can gradually and safely strengthen a weak back and neck.

**3. A variety of colors in our diet:** these different colors are nutrients and this variety of colors helps give us good complexion and skin tone as well as a broad spectrum of nutrients to supply our body with the tools it needs to work properly.

**4. Rapid and explosive movement:** though it may be the same amount of weight or distance, rapid and explosive movement builds muscle, as well as muscle, tendon, ligament, and bone strength.

**5. Build up of visceral (belly) fat:** a build up of fat around the organs can hold stored toxins that can leach into our organs poisoning their performance and longevity. Having an antioxidant rich diet from fruits and vegetables along with plenty of water and exercise helps safely lower the fat in this area and flush out these toxins.

**6. Aerobic exercise vs. Anaerobic exercise:** doing resistance circuit training, exercising large muscle groups gives both strengthening and cardiovascular benefits without wasting so much of your time. Remember these 3: Rapid – Explosive - Continuous Movement.

**7. Controlling sugar spikes:** controlling sugar spikes controls fatty deposits. Eating sugary and starch loaded foods prior to a sedentary period is like putting jet fuel in an idling engine.

**8. Breaking the Fast:** breakfast for most of us breaks approximately a 7-8 hour fast. We determine the type of fuel our body wants to burn throughout the rest of the day. Eating a high sugar breakfast will leave us craving sugar from the high levels of insulin in our blood simply from what we chose to eat in the morning. A sugary or carbohydrate loaded breakfast is like high octane fuel that burns out rapidly and dies, while protein, fat and complex carbohydrates are like logs that continue to emit a steady heat for hours!

**9. Sports conditioning and lifestyle conditioning:** are both about empowering functional movement and endurance. When you increase your strength and endurance for whatever your lifestyle functions and needs are, you enhance your performance and your quality of life.

**10. Keys to unleashing your inner pharmacy: 1.** Am I getting fresh air? **2.** Am I drinking 1/2 my body weight in ounces of water? **3.** Have I been eating healthy foods from the different food groups? **5.** Am I staying at the proper weight? **6.** Am I getting adequate rest? **7.** Am I getting plenty of sunshine? When we do the above with consistency, it strengthens a system that is like a personal doctor at work within us 24 x 7x 365 days a year that knows exactly what is wrong and what to do to fix it!

**11. Water retention:** you can decrease the amount of extra water your body feels it should retain by drinking more of it. It does this through the reverse process of arginine vasopressin.

**12. Water is a free fat burner:** calories are units of heat, so when we drink cold water, our body burns calories to warm up the water to your normal body temperature.

**13. Fat burning environment:** surround yourself with a variety of food choices that contribute toward your goals in health and fitness, get rid of the ones that undermine your goals.

**14. Do not stay low calorie for too long:** your body will think you're starving and it will reset your metabolism lower to survive the lower calorie schedule. An occasional binge meal helps reset your metabolism during extended periods of calorie restriction.

**15. Economy of movement:** when you strengthen your musculature to handle whatever you want or need to continue to do in life, you enhance your quality of life.

**16. Adding muscle and muscle strength:** lightens the load that is otherwise pulling and hanging on joints and skeletal structure.

**17. Your liver is your reserve snack machine:** we as a society are simply overstocking it with unburned sugars and high fructose corn syrup that is then converted to fat which then causes fatty livers and too much fat in our arteries and network of blood vessels.

**18. Personal responsibility:** when we are diagnosed with something, we should learn everything we can about it. It is through this knowledge that we are less apt to accept it as an ongoing condition that we keep on medicating without changing our lifestyle...

**19. Medication and Supplementation:** we need to know and personally understand why we are needing a medication or dietary supplement and if we need to stay on it, we need to understand this as well. When we understand our problem we are more apt to become proactive with changing lifestyle habits that oft times created this need in the first place.

A quote I really like and I believe can help us with whether or not we need to continue a medication or supplement is this: "Ask why, and ask it again five more times until all the artifice is stripped away and you end up with the intellectually honest answer."
~ Andy Grove

**20. The System:** setting health and fitness goals for 2014 can be great, but remember putting a system in place that you stick with is what gets you to your goals!

Remember, staying healthy, strong and having good mobility helps keep us independent from becoming dependent on a system that is growing increasingly unreliable!

# Keeping Health And Fitness Simple

We probably all know that our purchasing confusion tends to fatten someone else's pockets and empty ours, health and fitness is no different, in that confusion of what we need to do to stay or to get in shape often gets us to spend money for results we want with a solution someone else offers. This is what oft times drives sales in health, fitness, as well as the medical industry.

I've never been able to figure out why regular academics are taught in the final months of the senior's year in high school, when two of the most important things in a seniors life ahead are avoiding financial and health pitfalls, but then the financial and healthcare industries along with their shareholders wouldn't benefit from having several

100 million consumers making wise choices in their health and finance choices, would they?

Gym memberships, home exercise equipment and nutritional supplementation can be a great gap filler, but one of the fallacies of this industry's marketing ploys (for the potential consumer) is to give a person the feeling that they have to have what they offer to reach their health and fitness goals. The problem with this is that it provides too many excuses for a person that feels they cannot afford these solutions. Since when did eating less, eating healthy, burning stored energy/body fat, and staying active become something we think we HAVE TO pay someone else for? Activity, hydration, recovery and a balanced diet along with calorie control are the basic needs for health and fitness lifestyle, and this isn't an expensive to do list.

Why is it that we have more fat burners, nutritional products, and advanced medicine then in the history of this country, but we're fatter and unhealthier with more death from chronic disease then ever in our history as well? Could it be that we have become addicted to treating symptoms instead of showing our body we give a hoot about what its trying to do for us naturally and applying the lifestyle changes it so desperately wants us to make?

**Our body does not ask for much but it craves:** Clean air, Water, Balanced diet, Sunshine, Activity, Rest and wants us to slow down on the food intake when we're less active and increase it when we are active. Most of what any health, fitness or pharmaceutical business tries to provide for is simply a shortage or imbalance of the above! It is no different then a car that runs low in oil, uneven tire pressure, not enough engine coolant, stopped up air filter, using bad fuel, or simply letting it set still for too long. It's simple, the peak performance, life of the engine and life of the power train depends largely on how we use it and what we give it to consume.

**Challenge:** lets learn why we need clean air, water, balanced diet, sunshine, activity, rest, and learn why we need to slow down on food intake when we're less active and an increase when we are. When we learn why we need the above, we also learn what happens if we don't. This makes these healthy habits become much more important to us.

**Inexpensive fitness tips:**

**1.** If you cannot afford nutritional supplementation to bridge the nutritional gap in what you're getting through food, get a wide variety of colors in your diet.

**2.** If you cannot afford a gym membership or home exercise equipment, learn some body weight exercises that activate a lot of muscles into working together to create the movement, this helps make you more physically functional as well as stimulating an increase in cardio pulmonary activity.

**3.** Drink the cheapest drink with the highest value WATER!

When we really understand not only what our body needs, but why it needs it, a prescription for health starts to formulate and we can apply a lifestyle change that works like a designer medicine for not only what went wrong but also to increase our body's capabilities to prevent illness, disease and premature aging!

# Detoxing Our Body
# For Fat Loss!

How good would the inside of our house look and feel if everything was arranged neat as a button but was left really dirty. We would not feel complete (even if on surface things looked good) if we knew dust and filth were trapped in-on-around-and in-between fixtures, floors and the walls of our home. We know that keeping the environment inside our home clean helps keep the internal environment healthy. Our body should be treated no differently as we reorganize how our body is shaped and conditioned! If we don't detoxify our body and its systems, this toxic matter will be left in a more concentrated form (especially when we lose weight) since fat works like mucous in that it shields us from the toxin(s) it wraps itself around.

These toxins cause chronic inflammation when our body's vital organs, skin etc. get exposed to them, especially at higher concentrations! Decreasing body fat is great, but keep in mind that detoxing as you lose these protective layers is very important in guarding against premature aging and disease caused by inflammation and oxidative damage. Often along with rapid weight loss we see a person looking older with saggy skin and muscle tone. Getting to the proper weight and musculature is supposed to rejuvenate us and help us to look and feel younger not age us and increase our risk factor to disease!

**There are several ways to detox:** by doing a complete system cleanse and, or by simply having a diet rich in antioxidants and fiber from fruits and vegetables. I will address the two individually so you will know which one or combination would work best for you.

**1. Complete System Cleanse:** this usually references to a detox and cleanse of the liver, kidneys and colon. There are a lot of good ones available, but one I really like is a 7 Day system cleanse that comes with a list of foods to eat while using the cleanse. Many times it will eliminate 6-10+ pounds of waste from the midsection area (intestinal track), thus having a waistline sliming effect. Because of the typical American diet, many of us hold 10-20 pounds of waste that is not properly eliminated and this causes a swollen waist area. This is some very good weight to get rid of!

**2. Select a list of foods good for detoxing:** we should keep at least some of these foods in our diet every day to keep the level of toxins from building up in our body. Fruits and vegetables supply a load of antioxidants into our bloodstream that help remove toxins. Toxins cause oxidation and antioxidants help remove these things that cause oxidation, (btw oxidation causes rusting on vehicles so you can imagine what this means for our body when there is a lot of oxidative damage happening).

Eating only fruits and vegetables (at least 1/2 of them raw) will move all kinds of junk out within 5-7 days. Eat your fruits in the AM and vegetables in the PM, it works best with your body's natural detox cycle.

**Detox item list:** lemons, grapefruit, tart cherries, avocados, artichokes, asparagus, beets, broccoli, cauliflower, spinach, collard greens, kale, olive oil, coconut oil, cilantro, green tea, cabbage, garlic, ginger, turmeric, watercress, wheatgrass, milk thistle (great for liver) and last but most important WATER!!!

**We can assist our body's natural detox:** through sweat, plenty of water for a good urine elimination process, plenty of fiber for bile and food waste removal along with keeping our liver healthy so that it can continue to break down and metabolize toxic products and cholesterol out of our blood and into our body's waste basket for elimination from our body!

# Sugar Makes You Fatter Then Fat!

I've been saying for years that the two words I feel have been the most damaging in the obesity epidemic are "FAT FREE." If it's fat free and still tastes really good, you can bet it's loaded with sugar and if its sugar and fat free and doesn't pretty much taste like cardboard it's loaded down with chemical sugar substitute(s). With all the advice to eat low fat for the past 25+ years, why are we so fat???

Sugar spikes cause insulin surges and insulin promotes fat storage. Our body is only doing its job when it carts away extra sugars out of our blood and stores them in our fat cells. If our insulin does not lower our blood glucose to safe levels, things will become a sticky mess, leading to a host of problems such as poor circulation and blindness.

When we hear of or experience insulin insensitivity, diabetes and obesity, most of it is caused by making the choice to eat or drink sugar and starch products ahead of or after periods of inactivity, either way our body's capability to burn off this jet fuel properly is not there.

Naturally occurring fats in our foods are not the problem, (eggs, nuts, meats, avocados, coconuts etc.) but when we consume these fats and then dump sugars over a high fat meal or snack and get a spike in insulin, it changes the physiology of digestion leading to increased fat storage. We could probably put a big dent in the obesity epidemic by not drinking sweet beverages or desserts with our meals...

Food getting broken down into glucose is fuel to our body and if we eat foods that break down slower, our energy levels will stay steady without the highs and lows that come with high starch/sugar meals and snacks.

Another benefit when we start replacing high sugar foods (especially the processed ones) with healthy unprocessed foods is our calorie intake yields a higher level of nutrients, and these nutrients help us feed lean muscle and vital organs for a better shape and vitality, this helps us fight disease as well!

 Large amounts of sugar also kill off intestinal flora and we need the good bacteria from this gut flora to help stimulate the production of immune cells which in turn help break down bad toxic things in our diet that might cause us to get sick. Detoxing from refined sugars helps boost our immune system's capabilities!

 There are a few dietary changes we can make that can assist, double and even triple the progress in our fitness goals and one of the main ones is sugary food or drink (especially prior to or after periods of inactivity).

 Through the years I have seen many really hit their exercise routines hard, but the ones that double and triple the results they get, are the ones that watch what they consume! One 20 oz. soda or sweet tea would take around 45 minutes to walk off

**Reasons to curb usage of sugary food and drink:** aids in weight loss, helps control blood sugar and insulin levels, increased energy, more nutrient rich foods when sugary foods are replaced, improves immunity, reduces inflammation and risk of disease, less gas, battling fewer food cravings, better skin tone, and sharper mental clarity. Not sure how you feel, but the above list makes lowering sugar intake sound like a good idea!

**Remember:** if you want to keep sugar from making you fat; don't use it before or after periods of inactivity or low levels of activity, (it's like putting jet fuel in an idling engine)!

# Telomeres...Your Cellular Assembly Line

We are made up of several trillion cells and though we don't completely die as a person when several billion cells die in our body we can feel it in other areas such as low energy levels, sickness and chronic disease, as well as a loss of skin elasticity and other signs of premature aging.

Telomeres are the part of our cells that are like the end caps on shoe strings that keep the strings (DNA) from unraveling. As these end caps get wore down from new generations of cells passing through, we show first the signs of aging and eventually we come to the end of our life when too many of these telomeres get shortened to the point where they can no longer birth the new cells that rejuvenate us.

Studying this process seems a little complicated but it has helped me picture what happens better, when I imagine our telomeres being like an assembly line that assembles a product (new cells). If this assembly line got shorter each cycle, the end products would not come out looking as good as when they went through the full assembly line and eventually when the assembly lines are completely worn down, production stops and the factory shuts down.

Inside the several trillion cells of the body our DNA holds a blueprint of how it wants the next generation of cells to look like, and depending on how strong or how weak the assembly line is, determines how well the new generation of cells mirror the blue print of the parent cells. This assembly line is our lifestyle habits that can either help produce a healthy generation of cells or that can further corrode and damage this next generation of cells, causing premature aging and disease! This can also happen to the original blueprint (DNA) if it suffers from oxidative damage.

Have you ever noticed how some people carry much the same appearance throughout much of their adult life, while others do not look like the same person after the 30-40 years? Our external environment, and lifestyle habits have a lot to do with how our internal environment is set up for future generations of cells. This is why a person who has had premature aging (due to smoking, alcohol, drugs as well as inactivity, unhealthy or unbalanced diet, lack of sunshine, rest and other bad lifestyle habits) can oft times correct the above and gradually become younger in appearance along with an increase in vitality and energy.

There is new research that indicates that the enzyme telomerase can gradually rebuild the length of our telomeres and though they are uncertain as to whether it will extend cell life, they seem to be certain that it will extend the youthfulness of our new generations of cells vs. creating older decrepit cells. Either way lifestyle habits seem to be the leading factor of determining how we extend youthfulness into our latter years.

It can help us if we imagine our lifestyle habits as employees standing along our personal cellular assembly line building our next generation of cells. This assembly line will determine how they will look in appearance along with their capability to rejuvenate and fight disease! We can either employ bad habits or good habits...

**Assembly line employees that need to be FIRED:**

**1.** Polluted oxygen (smoking and other environmental toxins).

**2.** Processed Fluids (such as sodas and juices).

**3.** Unhealthy or unbalanced diet.

**4.** Lack of sunshine.

**5.** Inactivity.

**6.** Lack of good deep sleep.

**Hire these assembly line employees:** we can do this by identifying and replacing our bad habit(s) above with these...

**1.** Clean air.

**2.** Water.

**3.** Balanced diet from unprocessed foods.

**4.** Sunshine.

**5.** Exercising and staying active.

**6.** Deep-sleep and NO caffeine for 6 hours prior to sleep.

These employees of good health have synergy with each other and when one of the above employees are missing for a while or are not at work, it will show up in how you look, act and feel both physically and mentally!

**Remember:** you are made up of new cells every year, your healthy habits today determines your cellular make up for tomorrow!

I believe 100% that God designed our body with innate capabilities that no man has ever been able to match in modern medical science along with a unique capability to take the simple basics above and yield great health results.

# Which Type of Exercise
# Is Best For Me?

Aerobics, Strength Training, Plyometric training, Body Building, Cross Fit, Home Exercise Routines, Functional Training, Sports Conditioning, HIIT (high intensity interval training) and the list goes on and on. This list continues to grow whenever someone puts a new twist on something that is 1000's of years old.

The best thing someone can remember is that it all boils down to constrained physical activity that done over time builds strength, endurance, physique, metabolism, a better shape and a body that has cardiovascular and muscular capabilities to handle increased external forces both expected and unexpected.

Knowing the above can help make so we don't waste time or money in our pursuit of fitness. If we can simply find out what our individual need is, finding the right exercise program is as easy as finding the right piece to a puzzle.

**Types of exercise:** there are 2 primary ones; aerobic and anaerobic, then there's a combination of the two- aerobic and anaerobic. And if you want a combination of the two, get off the cardio equipment after your blood is warmed up, (do strength building exercises) and simply workout at a rapid pace working your large muscle groups. This builds strength and cardio endurance.

1. **Aerobic (cardio) exercise:** is primarily done for endurance, burning body fat and some muscle tone. These exercises are usually ones that are easy enough to do that an individual can continue for a longer period triggering the burning of body fat as energy and in achieving greater cardiovascular endurance.

2. **Anaerobic exercise (muscle building):** is simply an increase in resistance and though we cannot last as long doing it as its aerobic exercise counterparts, these exercises lead to muscle

strengthening, shaping, building and conditioning.

3. **Combining the two (cardio and strength training):** this is the line that I've been trying to blur for a long time and is simply done by exercising more rapidly using free weights and machines, or if doing bodyweight exercises, doing them more rapidly or explosively, (this gives more resistance to the exercise causing greater muscular stimulation during an otherwise aerobic only routine). The longer you are able to go without rest, the more your exercise is aerobic in nature, however the heavier or more restricted movements that decrease the time in any given set will make it more anaerobic in nature.

**Example:** if you were to carry a set of 5 lb. dumbbells up and down a driveway 10 times, your routine would be more endurance building (aerobic), as you increase your dumbbell weight you may be able to only do it 5 rounds which would be a combination of strength and endurance training, and if you increase it enough so you are able to carry the weight up the drive only one time, it will turn it into a anaerobic (strength building exercise).

**Finding the best program:** when we're looking to incorporate an exercise routine into our life, we should look simply at our lifestyle specific needs. This can be applied to strengthening and conditioning of an athlete, wanting to become swimsuit ready, or simply a senior that is wanting to be able to better handle his or her activities of daily living (ADL's). When we know what we want to strengthen in our life or what void we need to fill, selecting the right exercise program is no different then selecting the right supplement for a dietary deficiency.

Keep it simple and simply demand more from your exercise routine then you expect to confront in the real world and you will discover (besides your physical appearance), that whatever your day requires of you, will no longer take such a toll on you. This applies to elite athletes and extends to a senior simply looking to increase or maintain mobility and independent in the activities of daily living!

We all know what happens if we don't put the proper mix of ingredients together that a recipe calls for...it simply will not yield the desired outcome we were looking for.

# Hypertrophy Your Capabilities!!!

The goal for most of us (when exercising) is to strengthen, add shape to, enlarge or simply maintain our muscle(s) and their capabilities. Increasing muscle size and capability happens through a process known as hypertrophy, and is simply a muscle cell increasing in size and strength due to an increased demand we place on it.

The various types of muscle fibers will increase their capabilities depending on how we work them whether slow and long durations, or shorter, more powerful bursts when working them. Example: sprinting vs. jogging, using a set of 5 lb. dumbbells vs. 20 lb. Shorter durations with heavier weights (resistance) produce more strength and size while less weight and sets with longer durations has less strengthening effect but a more cardiovascular effect.

Our bone density, along with muscle, heart and lung strength responds in proportion with what we ask of it. Atrophy (shrinkage) whether in our muscle or our bones is oft times caused simply by a lack of use. Our body is not working purposely against us by shrinking our muscles and decreasing our bone density, it's just sizing us down to match us with our daily surroundings and what is required of it.

A very neat thing about our body though, is that it can rapidly pump up shrunken un-toned muscle that we used to have once we start using it in ways it used to be used. Muscle cells that used to be in good condition do not take long to come back. This is why after about 1-2 weeks you can see and feel muscle tone coming back in the areas that you exercise, if you don't believe it, try exercising only one bicep for several weeks and watch what happens.

Many of our arthritic conditions can be remedied by building muscle strength around these areas. If we looked at the different components of our musculoskeletal system (muscle, bones, ligaments, tendons, joints and bursa) as partners that rely on each other to carry out their individual duties and when the muscle side isn't strong enough to carry its own weight properly, it causes our weight to sag and hang from our skeletal structure. This causes more pressure on our tendon and ligament areas and if this continues we will have pain from chronic inflammation around our joint areas. Our muscle is a partner with our skeletal system and if it doesn't carry its share of the weight, it's going to upset the bones, joints, bursa, tendons and ligaments!

**Hypertrophy/muscle conditioning helps:**

**1.** Strengthen skeletal movement and capabilities.

**2.** Helps give our body shape.

**3.** Increases metabolism (toned muscle burns lots of calories).

**4.** Increased bone density, (our muscles tugging action on our bones, increases bone density).

**5.** Helps strengthen internal organs and other internal physiological processes.

**6.** Helps shield and protect vulnerable areas such as the nerves in our spinal cord.

**7.** Can help relieve the load on weight bearing joints and the list goes on and on!

The two primary ways to offset physical atrophy is through activity/exercise and dietary intake!

**Atrophy** = shrinking of muscle, tone and decrease physical capabilities.

**Hypertrophy** = increased muscle and physical capabilities.

We have the capability to strengthen or to weaken our body's God given capabilities by our own action or inaction!

# Strong Hearted

February is heart month and besides raising awareness for heart disease and prevention, the heart also gets to be the symbol for Valentines Day and weekend!

The month of February is used to bring attention to Heart Disease (the number one leading killer of American men and women) and to bring new research as well as prevention to the front lines. A lot of prevention advice centers around changing our dietary intake and increasing activity/exercise.

Despite the fact that approximately 25% of the population is on statin drugs and though dietary education has been aimed at eating low fat to decrease our risk, more Americans are dying then ever before from heart disease. And if you add in death from stroke, it seems the ticking time bomb we once spoke about is no longer ticking.

I would really like to see us here in our area, to start building a personal and community lifestyle that slows down the progression of this disease that is not only leading to premature aging and risk of death by heart attack and heart disease but is changing the natural sequence of death among people as well. When in history have we seen so many young people dying before their parents?

We can do things to help our hearts to become strong as well as keeping our network of blood vessels throughout our body healthy, flexible, elastic and clear of gunk that slows down the flow of nutrients the heart is trying to deliver to the different parts of the body. This can help alleviate blood pressure problems due to the simple fact that the heart can pump the blood through our network of blood vessels easier.

There are 3 primary habits that can help build a strong heart and a healthy system of blood vessels:

1. **Diet**

2. **Rest**

3. **Exercise**

**Dietary intake:** by increasing our intake of fruits, vegetables, nuts, beans and other antioxidant, fiber rich foods, along with fatty fish we can decrease inflammation and cholesterol throughout our vascular system and decrease the fat in our liver.

Inflammation causes cholesterol to build up in our blood vessels, decreasing the flow of oxygen and nutrient rich blood from reaching their points of destination. Cholesterol is very much needed as a nutrient in the body, but very detrimental to vascular health if it sticks to the walls of our blood vessels instead of getting to their cellular destination.

Drink plenty of water! If our blood plasma levels drop due to a dehydrated or partially dehydrated state, our heart has to work much harder to pump the lessor volume of blood. When our heart rate starts increasing for no other known reason such as excitement, exercise or activity, chances are we may be dehydrated. Drink half of your bodyweight in ounces of water.

**Exercise:** exercising all parts of the body helps circulate blood throughout our body's network of blood vessels and helps build a strong heart muscle that will in turn help it pump blood much easier to parts of the body that are or become active. Steady exercise (continued movement) for at least 30 minutes helps increase our nitric oxide levels, which helps our blood vessels and helps with hypertension and blood pressure problems.

**Rest:** deep rest and relaxation helps repair, recharge, de-stress and rejuvenate a heart, mind and body! Deep rest and recovery helps our body's vital organs and systems to handle the demands placed on them and help us keep them younger. Don't intake a caffeinated or stimulant product less then 6 hours prior to sleep.

Researching heart disease and heart healthy diets is something we should do individually and as a community, this can help us find the lifestyle offsets to give our heart the tools it needs to fight the battles it oft times is silently struggling inside our chest to win for you and me. I hope you stay strong hearted!

# Free Natural Fat Burners

Most fat burners and legitimate weight loss guidelines are designed to enhance your thermogenic state, so that more of your stored fat is being broken down into a syrupy brown substance to be burned as energy or as a source of calories for the days that you don't eat enough to cover your body's daily calorie use.

I've listed several ways below that you can naturally light up the fat burning state in your body and one cheap way (at the end of the article) that you can increase thermogenic activity (fat burning) throughout your exercise routine using a combination of two items you probably already have in your cabinets.

**Temporary food restriction:** When we drop our calories really low for 1-2 days or fast for 18-24 hours, it will create a calorie deficit. Our body will pull calories from our stored fat to give us the fuel we need to cover our daily energy requirements, (a pound of stored fat will yield around 3500 calories). This is why we lose weight when we either drop our calorie intake or skip eating for 18-24 hours. You don't want to do this for too long or your body will sense starvation and will begin breaking down your most metabolically active tissue (muscle) to slow down your metabolism. The trick is in getting your calorie intake back up before this process starts. If you use fat burners to curb your appetite, get off of it every 3-4 days to let your appetite return.

**Temperature control:** temperature control is one of the biggest calorie burners we have going on in our body. Our body is constantly trying to regulate our temperature whether its to warm us or cool us down, this activity burns a lot of calories! Whether its in the heat of the summer and our body is trying to expel heat or if its in the cold of winter and our body is shivering to create heat and using up calories which are units of heat, our external environment can cause our body to burn a lot of calories just to regulate internal environment.

Recently we had an extended cold snap and my electrical energy usage almost doubled, our body is much the same especially when it's keeping our body around 98.6 F and the external temperature is 30-60 degrees cooler. This is why our appetite sometimes surges in the winter. This is also a good time to force the body to release body fat when lower our calorie intake and we enhance this capability by not eating anything sweet as a source of the calories we eat, (sweet foods temporarily block the body's capability to release fat for energy).

**Digestion of food:** Our food choices can cause our body to burn more calories during digestion because of a thing called the thermic effect of food. Not all calories are the same, some absorb very rapidly into our system causing a spike in blood sugar and other foods have to go through more of the digestive process to break down, causing us to burn more calories throughout the digestion process.

**Example:** chicken breast, serving of broccoli, and sweet potato vs. a milk shake. It doesn't take much effort to digest the shake and with the rapid absorption comes increased potential of the extra fuel in our blood being carted off and stored in our fat cells.

**Cheap thermogenic enhancer:** take an aspirin about 15-30 minutes prior to a workout and drink a cup of coffee just before your workout, you can almost feel your fat cells releasing their energy!

Stored fat is like work we've done in advance...its stored food that we've already ate, processed and stored. It sets there ready to be used when we don't have time to eat or when we feel we need to get rid of some of the excess groceries in our pantries.

# Inflammation ÷ Pain and Disease = Billions$$$

There is probably no other physical issue that costs our society as much hardship, pain and money then inflammation. We would probably pay a lot more attention to inflammation if we would more strongly associate how large a part it plays in pain, premature aging, disease and death.

Acute inflammation is a healthy part of our immune system and helps with the healing process in a traumatized area. Chronic inflammation happens when this process doesn't get shut down properly (due to continued aggravation to this area or an outside invader such as too many vaccinations, continued use of antibiotics, bad air, or food components that aggravate our digestive tract and ones that our body cannot process properly and eliminate).

Chronic inflammation's continued smoldering will eventually manifest itself as a disease wherever it's at and depending on its behavior will spread to other parts of the body.

This can happen to our brains as well from a continuously artificially stimulated immune system. I personally think it weird that we give our babies 5-20 vaccinations between birth and 5 years of age and think the immune/inflammatory response will not affect the organ in their head.

We need to ask ourselves why after 1000's of years are we suddenly encouraged to use all sorts of vaccinations, why are 1 in 80 of our children are autistic, why has there been a 400% increase in antidepressant usage, why are so many needing to be on brain control drugs as they get older (to keep them from nutting up on themselves or society), why do Americans consume 80% of the worlds pain meds later in life, why do our governing bodies piously fight this massive war on drugs (that are responsible for far fewer deaths) while putting their stamp of approval on ones that cause lots of death &

changes in behavioral patterns, why has chronic disease exploded in the past 40 years? Could it be that we have an INFLAMMATION NATION and the causes of inflammation are being looked away from with a focus on symptoms only?

If most all chronic disease comes from inflammation and most anything that effects our body is from things we either breath in, consume, or inject we have to look no further then this if we really want to figure it out.

Treating the various ways inflammation prevails itself, cancers, heart disease, brain disorders, digestive problems etc. has developed into a huge industry and if the inflammation starts to disappear, so does this band aide industry's profits.

**Acute inflammation:** this is the initial puffiness surrounding an injured, or traumatized area and is a healthy part of our immune system and part of the recovery process.

**Chronic inflammation:** is simply when the above does not turn off properly, or if something continues to trigger an immune/inflammatory response over a lengthened period of time, it then becomes the potting soil for the seed of disease, whether brain, muscular, skeletal or our vital organs.

Inflammation can be chronic joint inflammation prevailing itself as arthritic conditions, inflamed blood vessels stiffening and causing vascular/heart disease, as well as organs of the body eventually having a cancer named after them once inflammation has been there long enough such as pancreatic, lung, liver or esophageal cancer. Most times when the inflammation in a particular area gets a name it has had something happening to it for a long time and it has finally come to a boiling point. It's at this point that it can be diagnosed and named after the body part it's originating from.

**Pain Therapy tip:** most chronic pain stems from inflammation and if you can find the site the inflammation is at, cool it down with an ice pack and if you don't have an ice pack, use a cold pack of rice. Take an anti-inflammatory such as Ibuprofen. The idea is to shrink down the puffiness of the inflammation in the area the problem is stemming from, thus lessening the pressure on nerves in this area.

Finding the source of inflammation is like retreating back down a trail to find where you took a wrong turn.

# Weight Loss and Aging

I think we would all agree that healthy weight loss is the best weight loss, but many of us fall in that trap of waiting too long and then being in a hurry to lose weight and wind up doing it in a way that can potentially age our physical appearance as well as our vital organs.

Over the years I have seen the difference many times that a healthy weight loss makes in rejuvenating and revitalizing a person's appearance vs. unhealthy weight loss that results in a saggy aged appearance due to a loss of muscle tone and a decrease in nutrients that keeps us healthy.

This aged appearance that we see on the outside is indicative of what's going on inside as well.

**Here's why:** when we have a sustained drop in calories over too long a period, far below the amount our body burns per day, our body detects starvation and starts breaking down muscle to burn as fuel. This usually starts after about 3-4 days of low caloric intake and is a natural defense mechanism in helping us avoid dying from starvation, and since muscle burns a lot more calories then fat, decreasing our muscle helps slow our metabolism down so that we can get by on fewer calories. Most times we can see if this is happening because of a gaunt tired, aged appearance. This is due to protein breakdown and will cause skeletal weakness, loss of muscle tone and skin elasticity as well as a weakening of our organs since they are made of protein as well.

Protein breakdown doesn't mean that your skeletal muscles or your vital organs are going to quit working; they will simply become weaker, less efficient and age prematurely.

When we use fat burners etc. that curb our appetite, we need to get off them every 3-4 days and increase our calorie intake. This restocks the skeletal muscle, vital organs and other parts of the body with fuel, after this it is safe once again to drop calories back down, especially on non-workout days. Zigzagging your calorie intake is a trick way to get your body to release calories stored in your fat cells, thus shrinking them.

 Following this zigzag approach to calorie intake will help avoid the decrease in metabolism (loss of muscle) as well as helping rejuvenate your body instead of aging you!

 Whenever you create a draw down on your fat cells, you should increase antioxidant intake (fruits and vegetables) and water to help flush the toxins out. Our body uses fat cells and mucous to protect us from toxins and when we lose fat too rapidly without helping our body detox, these toxins can come into our body's systems and cause aging and other chronic issues. Fruit is great for detoxing and since our body is in a detox state for approximately 6 hours after waking up, this time period is a good time for fruit.

 **Tip:** On low calorie days, completely cut out sugars and starches. This lowers the insulin in your blood and helps trigger the release of calories from your fat deposits. Fatty deposits are simply stored calories for periods of food shortage.

Building muscle and tone is how we build or rebuild our metabolism, this turns you into the burner of fat instead of every year feeling that you have to buy more fat burners to artificially stimulate your thermogenic activity!

# Mood Shape-Up!

There is a very good perk that comes with an exercise routine whether its for shapeup, strengthening, athletics, or mobility, this perk is a release of endorphins that simply make us feel good and help us get rid of brain stress that can put stress on our body and its functions.

Doing intense periods of activity/exercise regularly helps keep us strong in mind, body and spirit and besides the euphoric feeling exercise gives, it can also help lessen the perception of pain, and even works as a sedative. These endorphins bind to some of the same neuron receptors that pain medicine binds to, to block pain signals. Exercise is simply one of the best ways to ease anxiety and stress, but unlike pain pills, antidepressants and anxiety drugs, it has awesome side effects!

Now for the interesting part, I would like to list some of the things that happen with continued use of exercise and then a list of what can happen with continued use of pain medicine and medications for depression...

**Exercise:** reduces stress, wards off anxiety and feelings of depression, boosts self-esteem, improves sleep, improves energy levels, increases physiological functions such as regularity, water and temperature control, better cardiopulmonary circulation, strengthens heart, lowers blood pressure, increased libido, improves muscle tone, shape and strength, builds bone density, builds tendon, ligament and joint strength as well as joint lubrication, helps reduce body fat, helps build an increased metabolism, okay I'll stop now...

**Pain medicine benefits and side effects:** blocks pain signals but oft times gives a drugged feeling of euphoria, cognitive effects on the brain, nausea, constipation, drug tolerance and dependence, stress on kidneys causing urinary difficulty, skin itchiness and dryness, slows down central nervous system, and can have horrible effects on our liver (the organ that is responsible for over 500 functions in our body) and after all the above listed side effects, it is not a cure for what's actually causing the pain!

**Note:** many of the pain medicines when combined with alcohol are like drinking poison to the liver.

**Antidepressant benefits and side effects:** helps reduce depression, helps create a more positive feeling, can balance brain chemistry, but can increase a feeling of security in things one would've and possibly should've felt insecure with before, and can oft times cause an increased acceptance of how things are instead of a desire to create positive change for oneself and in the lives of others, can cause nausea, insomnia, drowsiness, lack of concentration, sweating, vomiting, dry mouth, diarrhea or constipation, dizziness, irritability, weight gain, sexual disturbances, and if suddenly discontinued can cause deep dark depression, explosive dangerous behavior either to ones self or others, suicidal thought and suicide, cause dependence on a drug for how we feel and view life, as well as adapting us to a lifestyle of medicating unhappiness and depression instead of getting off our rear ends and doing something about what is causing our unhappiness and depression!

When we look at the above listed pros and cons, it's not hard to figure out what we should be making a continuing part of our life and what we should not. I am not completely anti-drug use, but after using a drug (if needed) to intervene between us and the symptoms, but we should immediately start looking for the cause of the symptom and what lifestyle changes we can make to cure the problem instead of continuing to medicate the problem's symptoms!

Exercise and a good diet is like a lake with good inflows and out flows, and if this activity stops the water stagnates, good things die and bad things grow...

Exercise helps to release the body's natural pain inhibitors and the good feeling endorphins that God designed our body to produce naturally, the pharmaceutical industry simply formulates and intensifies synthetic products that attempt to duplicate what our body does naturally.

# Whole Food Nutrition vs. Supplements

Supplements are like a cane or crutch, if we don't have a weakness the cane or crutch is not necessary. If we can find the weakness in our diet, we can add in a supplement that can possibly yield a lot of health value for the money spent, but if we don't have a weakness or gap in our diet, its like using a crutch or splint when its not necessary, it might give us a feeling of security, but its doing more harm then good.

To bring common sense back into things, we need to look no further then what our body likes to use and the tools it needs for maintenance and good health. One of the primary things it needs to do this is whole food nutrition through a balanced diet that supplies proteins, fats, carbs, enzymes and micronutrients, from fruits, vegetables, and other plant life items along with probiotic rich foods.

**Whole food:** whole food is a food that has not been processed into a different form.
**Example:** an apple, not apple dumpling.

If we cannot go back through our diet over a few days and see a trail of nuts, berries, lean meats, cultured/fermented products, vegetables, fruits and beans, with water as a source of hydration, we have probably identified why we may not be feeling well! If our car started sputtering after a fill-up of fuel, how long would it take us to figure out that it might be the fuel?

For digestive nutrients, we need an adequate amount of raw foods (fruits and vegetables), cultured foods (yogurt, buttermilk, pickles, sauerkraut and cheese), these foods that contain probiotics, help replenish our digestive tract with enzymes that help us break foods down and extract their nutrients much better.

Whole food has 1000's of little unnamed nutrients: unlike vitamins that may have 30-60 named nutrients on their labels, fruits, vegetables, nuts, berries etc. have 1000's of named and unnamed nutrients that work together and absorb much better into our body. When our body has these 1000's of nutrients to choose from, it's like giving a mechanic a good set of tools to work with!

**Example:** I have a list of the named nutrients in an apple (there are 400 on this list) but it's said to be 1000's of unnamed nutrients in a single apple. We don't know why they are there, but the apple and all the other nutrients in the apple know why they are there. Imagine a band that has a full set of instruments going, it simply sounds better with a complete harmony of instruments bringing their individual unique sound to the stage. Now imagine how bad it would sound if only one individual band member and instrument showed up to do the job of many.

 **Supplements:** supplements are intended to fill the missing gap in our diets, a lot like a substitute band member on standby. However to think all supplements are equal is like thinking all substitute band members are the same. If you feel something is missing in your diet, and if you cannot increase this part of your diet through food, adding in a supplement to bridge the gap can be a good choice if it comes from a good company with a good track record.

**Example:** many of us do not get close to the daily intake of fruits and vegetables recommended by the CDC for prevention of chronic disease. In this case either increasing our intake of fruits and vegetables or taking a fruit and vegetable supplement can be a good choice. Another example of potential use of a supplement is if someone is working out regularly and needs more protein (and since muscle is made of protein) our body has an increased need for protein, in this case you could add a protein shake and or amino acids to fill in for this increased need. However, you can simply increase your intake of, meat, dairy, nuts, beans etc. and possibly get even better results.

One of my worst pet peeves is when someone fragments the nutrients from an egg to increase their protein intake by only eating the egg white and discarding the yolk. This part of the egg is loaded with nutrients and the egg white knows exactly why these nutrients are there, and why it can do a much better job in our body when its consumed together and not fragmented away from its origin.

If we could see the millions of actions and reactions that happen in our body, we would better understand its need to pick and pull from the 1000's of nutrients that nature provides through whole food nutrition that grows around us. The nutrients in whole food have a synergistic effect on each other and when consumed have an amplified effect in our body.

Do things that grow well and do well in our region, just maybe provide an answer for us as a person as well?

# The Value of Instability
# In Exercise

Our muscle's constant fight against instability strengthens and keeps our stabilizer muscles strong, enhancing our stability and balance!

This is something I've been thinking a lot about the past couple weeks since a friend of mine told me that her mother-in-law fell off the toilet because she could not hold herself up properly. My friend has been trying to get her to do things to increase her strength, but she simply has not wanted to do anything the past year except the minimal daily functions and her muscle has atrophied accordingly as well as her capability to stabilize.

When we are constantly supported by something, whether sitting, standing, walking and even exercise, our stabilizer muscles become weaker. This is a huge benefit that free weight and bodyweight exercises provide, due to our body having to stabilize the movement vs. a machine doing it for us. There are lots of little stabilizer muscles that engage to hold us steady and help pull us back into balance whenever we get off balance. When these muscles are not used regularly whether through exercise or through our daily activities, they simply become weaker and weaker.

Free weight and bodyweight exercise vs. machines: a benefit of free weight exercises and bodyweight exercises is they exercise muscle groups like we use them in daily life. When we are lifting, pulling or pressing something in our daily routine and even if we're just standing still unsupported by anything, our body is constantly trying to balance itself or the object that force is being put into. Machines on the other hand target the primary muscle groups but leave out many stabilizer muscles because the machine is doing the stabilization work for us. Another example of something that works stabilizer muscle and one that doesn't is a bicycle vs. a tricycle.

You can test how strong your stabilizer muscles in your legs are by trying 3 simple moves.

**1.** Spread your feet, lean forward, backwards, then side to side.

**2.** Next try to do the same thing with your feet tight together, (keep something close that you can grab hold of if you lose your balance).

**3.** Next hold on to something if you need to, but try to see how long you can stand on one foot.

There are so many things in life that try to throw us off-balance, that by simply living a very active lifestyle our balance improves due to the constant use of our stabilizer muscles against destabilization forces. So we're exercising our stabilizer muscles simply by being active! When we get inactive our muscles, tendons, ligaments and bones get weaker, but the capability to steady ourselves (or whatever our workload is) gets weaker as well.

**Stability exercise:** do a freestanding squat and as you come up thrust your arms upward toward the ceiling, you can use dumbbells in this movement as well. You can decrease your stability and force more stabilizer muscles to work by simply putting your feet together and doing the same movement, repeat movement as many times as you can for several sets after an initial warm up set.

Sometime while standing, move your feet tightly together and just stand there and feel all the little muscles twitching from your toes to your torso that are working to balance you and keep you from falling.

The gift of balance is one that goes away when left unchallenged...

# Nature's Farmacy

I've been an advocate for increasing fruit and vegetable consumption for years for prevention of disease and premature aging, so when I heard the announcement on CBS on April 1, 2014 about the European study that just came out, it was really exciting to me!

This study covered 65,226 participants ages 35+ for over 7 years and found a 42% reduction in risk of dying from common diseases in ones that ate at least 7 servings of fruits and vegetables a day. Additionally they reduced their risk for heart disease and cardiovascular complications by 31% and cancer risk by 25%.

Its simple, your choice of foods can lower or increase your risk of death by chronic disease! The Centers for Disease Control has for years been putting a push behind fruit and vegetable consumption for prevention of chronic disease, as well as it being important for optimal child growth and for weight management.

This is big when you know that the biggest killer of Americans is heart disease, 2nd is cancer, and the 3rd leading cause of death is medical misdiagnosis, hospital infections and pharmaceutical drug complications.

When we can lower our risk to the above by changing our food choices and adding in a few other healthy lifestyle habits, it simply increases our body's ability to prevent disease on its own and decreases its reliance on intervention by medicine and medical facility. There are billions $$$ made by the fear mongering of the masses to use invasive machines for early detection, when they're perfectly healthy. We should pay much more attention to what's causing the disease instead of early detection of it.

Spring is an exciting time of the year where seeds are sprouting, plants and trees are blooming with the beginnings of the loaded nutritional packets they will be working on over the next few months and bringing to us in the form of fruits, vegetables, nuts, beans and other whole foods. We should all try to grow something ourselves, whether its planting a tomato plant in a big flower pot, a few blueberry plants in a corner of the yard or whatever other fruit or vegetable we like. If its something we like, we'll probably enjoy watching it develop the food more.

Many of us either do not have the space or time to grow a large garden, but if we can increase the value of local grown fruits and vegetables by purchasing them, we will increase the demand and reward for the growers around us. We have a new thing that is starting here in Fort Valley called Veggies in the Valley, that will have 4 gardens managed by local gardeners here in the community. Hopefully this spawns a lot of individual gardens and gardeners in the coming years.

When we consume fruits and vegetables grown in our region, we increase the chances of them getting picked at the ripened stage when nature intended for it to be harvested. We don't like to work on a project for a long time only to have it taken from us before we're finished with it and neither does a plant, ever notice how hard it is to pull an un-ripened fruit or vegetable from its plant, but how easy it is when the plant is finished with it?

There are loads of antioxidants and fibers in fruits and vegetables that help detoxify our bodies. The antioxidants from fresh fruits and vegetables help get rid of toxic debris throughout our organs, skeletal structure as well as the fibers and plant enzymes that help us maintain a healthy digestive tract.

Energy and defense nutrients are in the foods that nature develops and our body can feel the difference whether in energizing us or in helping us fight illnesses as well as chronic and infectious diseases!

There is no one that can develop food better then nature itself!

# Calculating Calories

I think we have gotten a little off track in how we think that low calorie is always better, when the main reason we actually need to eat is for the calories. It's one of the most life sustaining items after oxygen and water. It's the excess over what we need that becomes fat (stored energy). We simply need to keep track of the times we consume to much, so that we can lower the amount we consume the next meal or the next day.

When we fill up our car with fuel, how soon we need to refuel is dependent on how much we use our car. Our body does have a lot going on inside, so whether we're active or just setting still, our body burns a large amount of calories just to maintain itself.

All the formulas, calculations and multiplication tables for our calorie needs, probably do a lot more for confusing us then if it were less accurate but easy to remember. If it wasn't for the low fiber content in much of the food we eat, we could trust our gut to tell us when we need more fuel or have enough. Fiber in our food is a little like a fuel control valve, without it, our system gets loaded with fuel causing what we know as sugar spikes.

To figure a close estimate of the amount of calories needed, simply calculate your ideal body weight x 10 and it will give you a close amount of what you need to support yourself at that weight if you're holding still.

**Example:** 150 lb. x 10 = 1500 calories a day.

**Next:** to figure out approximately how much you need for fueling your daily activities, simply multiply your base calorie need by .3, .4, .5, or .6 depending on how light or heavy your activity level is for the day. So if you have a very light day multiply .3 x 1500 = 450 for your extra activities need. 1500 + 450 = 1950. If you have a heavy day such as heavy manual labor, a long strenuous workout, or simply one of those non-stop days, multiply your base calories by .6.

**Using the example above:** 1500 x .6 = 900, which gives you an approximate need of 2400 calories for a heavy day.

You can get a more accurate amount by separating calories burned for digestion, but I like figuring it into the calories burned in daily activities to keep it easier.

Even though you need to aim to cover your daily calorie need, if you suddenly drop way below the amount your body normally burns in a day, it will temporarily trigger the release of stored fat. However if this goes on for too long your body will detect food shortage issues and survival mode will kick in to lower your metabolism and it does this by burning through muscle as a fuel source.

Following a zigzag pattern with your calorie intake, low calorie on inactive days and higher calorie on the active days is a trick way to burn body fat without the muscle loss that ages our body. Keeping starches and sugars low on the low calorie days is the key for releasing body fat for energy.

If you've got a smart phone, there are some really neat apps that can be downloaded that will do a lot of the calorie calculations and other monitoring work for you. My Fitness Pal is a really good one to download and learn how to use. It allows you to scan barcodes on foods for calorie content and to calculate your consumption for the day simply by entering activity levels.

Whichever way you decide to do it, remember that calories are simply the way our body fuels activity and whether its food calories we consume to meet our energy demands, or calories from stored body fat, our body is going to get it from somewhere. Its when we go low calorie for too long that we start breaking down muscle for fuel, and this is our body simply slowing the metabolism down to accommodate the new continuous low calorie schedule.

To lose weight simply drop calorie intake way down and eat only high fiber low sugar foods for about two days and your body will release calories from body fat, thus shrinking fat cell size.

# Medical Roulette

I hesitated about writing this one, because just like my uncle, aunt and many friends, there are many others in the medical field that are passionate, clear minded, responsible line backers in helping us fight the health care battles we come up against!

However, we should not turn a blind eye to an industry that has largely benefited from blind trust, which has helped medical misdiagnosis, hospital infections and adverse drug reactions become the 3rd leading killer behind heart disease and cancer.

**Journal of AMA April 15,1998:** The government is pushing medical care as healthcare, but the more prescriptions one takes, the worse someone's health becomes. Drugs create illness due to Adverse Drug Reactions that make medical care a leading cause of death. Adverse drug reactions are defined as "from a drug properly prescribed and administered." It's not an overdose or bad prescription. It's just the way that patient reacted unexpectedly.

**Centers for Disease Control (CDC) 2008:** More people die every year from prescription drug abuse than die from heroin and cocaine combined.

**Wall Street Journal Sept 21, 2012:** Medical errors kill enough people to fill four jumbo jets a week.

**USA Today April 16, 2014:** A USA Today review shows more than 100,000 doctors, nurses, medical technicians and health care aides are abusing or dependent on prescription drugs in a given year, putting patients at risk.

We have grown a reliance on an industry that is simply not sustainable. And until we can get back to where medicine and medical care facility is used as a tool for temporary intervention, this problem will probably get much worse! Using the awesome advancements in medicine is great for intervention, but we should STOP continuing to use these drugs so that we don't have to change the lifestyle that lead up to the problem in the first place. Have you ever done business with anyone that doesn't want returning customers?

**What we can do:** if we have a problem that is acute enough (that our body cannot recover on its own with corrected lifestyle habits) take the medicine to intervene between you and the symptoms. If it's a problem enough to take a medicine, then it's a problem enough to research where the health issue is originating. We can do this by understanding first what the medicine is for and then working our way backwards.

**Example self diagnosis:** if someone is overweight and gets put on blood pressure medicine, we should first look at what is causing the high blood pressure. If we think it is being overweight and too much dietary sodium, we should then find out what is causing us to be overweight and where the excess sodium is coming from, then make the necessary lifestyle changes in our life to get us back on track. In this case being overweight is very likely from lack of exercise and diet; the high sodium is probably from too many processed foods and or added salt.

To NOT research and fix where the problem is coming from and to choose to continue medicating it instead, is like having a leak in our house and being content to just put a bucket under the leak. The problem will later manifest itself in more destructive ways then just a wet floor, such as rotted wood, rusting and an overall aging of the structure we live in. In this case, suppliers of construction materials and carpenters are the ones that benefit from us not finding and stopping the leak.

The timelines above and statistics seem to be getting worse and it seems to be doing this in direct correlation with an increased dependence on others for our healthcare instead of personal responsibility. We see this in our healthcare system as well as our welfare system. We as an individual, family and community can change this by taking personal responsibility in the things blessings we should value.

Do others put more effort into my health and well being then I do myself?

# Real Life Value of the Pushup and Squat

Pushups and freestanding squats, will exercise muscle groups (or parts of muscle groups) that are often passed over if someone does not exercise regularly. Pushups and squats when doing the full range of motion will help activate the muscle fibers of these particular muscle groups.

I believe a lot of the back problems we have comes from us doing way more pulling then we do pushing (in our activities of daily living) and this creates muscle imbalances. A good way to know if your pushing muscles are conditioned is to see if the back of your upper arm is flabby or toned.

**Why the pushup works so well:** we don't use our pushing muscles as much as our pulling muscles and the muscles we use for pushing (when left unused) get untoned and flabby. The two primary muscle groups we use for pushing with our upper body is our chest and triceps muscles and the two spots we tend to begin to sag is the back of our arms (triceps) and our chest (pectoral) muscles.

**The 2nd reason:** it gets us into a similar position as the plank and engages our core, back and neck muscles in a static contraction as we're actively working our chest, shoulders, and triceps muscle groups throughout the pushup movement.

So not only is this working the entire chest area, shoulders, and back of the arms, it is also shaping and strengthening our midsection, back and neck muscles.

### Different forms of pushups:

**1.** The standard pushup where the only continuous contact with the floor is our hands and our toes/toe balls.

**2.** If the standard pushup is too hard, do the pushup where the knees are used as a secondary contact point with the toes.

**3.** If getting on the floor is too difficult or not practical, simply lean at a slant against something such as a table or railing. Lean into it, and then push yourself back in much the same way as a regular pushup.

**To increase resistance:** increase speed of movement or put a small stack of books under each hand when doing the regular floor pushup to increase the stretch, resistance and distance of the movement.

**Why the squat works so well:** we need the capability to pull ourselves back up if our knees ever buckle under us. When this happens we oft times realize how weak our leg muscles have become. Weak legs are like walking with stilts in that as long as they stay fairly straight, everything is fine, but if they ever get caught off balance, it can be almost impossible to correct back into an upright position. Squats strengthen the very muscles we need for standing up from a sitting position, getting back up from a squatting position as well as strengthening the muscles we need to help correct our balance when we stumble. If these muscles are really weak and our knees buckle, we tend to continue in a southern direction.

**Different ways to do the squat:**

**1.** Hold unto something and lower yourself into a squatting position. If your knees hurt, lean backwards with your feet almost up under whatever you are holding onto so that all your weight is on your heels, then slightly lift the front of your feet as you're going through the squatting movement. This will take the pressure off your knees and will really work the hamstrings and buttocks.

**2.** Regular standing squat. I like holding my hands out in front of me as I lower into a squat, then thrust them upwards when I come back up.

**Use good form:** keep your knees from going past your toes, (this keeps pressure off your knees). You simply want to squat the buttocks down in-between your heels like you would if you were squatting around a fire.

**There are two common ways of increasing power in the squat:** speed of movement and added resistance. Jump squats after an initial warm up, can help build and tone muscle. To do this movement, simply drop into a squat, and then explode upward reaching your arms upwards for a good core strengthening movement.

This works really well as a circuit exercise when you rotate from squats to pushups, since it works different muscle groups and while one group is resting, you're working the next group, thus keeping your heart rate up and stimulating increased lung activity. This helps turn your workout into a cardio, fat burning, and muscle-stimulating workout all in one!

The pushup strengthens the muscles that help lift us up off the floor and the squat strengthens muscles that help keep us from stumbling and hitting the floor.

# What Burpees and Falling Have In Common

It is something that is pretty sure to happen to us at one point or the other, the problem is it seems to be a lot harder to recover, as we get older. However if practice makes us better at doing things, would this not apply to falling as well?

As we get older we tend to get down on the floor or ground less often, and about the only time we're in a prone position is at an elevated position such as our bed, so the muscles used gradually shrink in size and strength as well as gradually lose capability to properly work with each other.

To get these muscles activated, toned, strengthened and the nerve communications working properly with each other, we simply need to practice getting in and out of this compromised position. There are several levels of intensity; start with whatever is light intensity for your physical condition.

**Athletic intensity:** this is not the proper terminology but is none the less what someone does when repeatedly and rapidly dropping to the floor into a prone position (like a pushup) then rapidly getting back up with a slight jump while reaching overhead. These are known as burpees and are very intense! Repeat this movement until tiring.

**Moderate intensity:** drop into a squatting position, then crawl forward on all fours, then lay prone on the floor, get back upright on your knees and then stand back up not using any support. Repeat several times.

**Light intensity:** same as above except for pressing your hand against thigh above knee area as a support lever when standing back up.

**Ultra light intensity:** stand beside a sofa (or something solid to hold onto) and lower yourself first down to the knees, then down into a prone position on the floor, then get back up on your knees and using the support of the sofa or other solid fixture, pull yourself back up into a standing position. Rest for a little and then repeat if able.

**Beginner therapy:** if you have had an injury or simply are to weak to do the above, don't give up this one will help give you a foundation to do the ultra light intensity one above. A lot of the same muscles are activated when we get out of our bed from lying in a prone position. Do this several times or until tiring, rest, and then repeat. Gradually you'll see this get easier and easier allowing you to move up to the next level as your body becomes more capable.

To increase strength in any one of the above, simply increase the speed of movement and increase the amount of repetitions. When this gets easy, move up to the next level of intensity.

The above movements are functional movements that we use in real life and they activate most of our skeletal muscle, so you will notice an increase in heart rate as well as heavier breathing, (working muscles need blood and oxygen) and since this activates a lot of muscle, it gives your heart and lungs a workout as well. If you do not believe you can get a good workout doing this, try doing any of the above 10 times without stopping. This is also a thermogenic fat burner exercise as well, because of the amount of muscles activated, especially when done rapidly.

There is no universal gym as unique to your specific needs as the human body itself!

# Last Minute Summer Shape-Up Tips

Spring is the time of year when I try to get members to calm down and realize they're not instant pudding. We simply cannot go high speed into size reduction without a loss in shape and this comes from the loss of muscle triggered by extended crash diets (that don't have regularly scheduled cheat meals).

I cannot stress it enough, if you want to shape up fast, simply build muscle tone underneath the body fat and gradually decrease body fat. Body fat does not look so bad if it has good skeletal muscle shape underneath. This looks much better then the smaller saggy shape (that comes with rapid weight loss) and it's much healthier too! And as your muscle builds up your metabolism will increase helping it become easier to shed unwanted body fat.

A common mistake many make is to get on an appetite suppressant/fat burner and go low calorie all the way to their goal weight, but once obtained look completely different then they used to at that same weight. The primary reason is a loss of muscle/protein in the body, and this is where the aged, saggy appearance comes from. This also causes a person's metabolism to drop due to all the muscle that was lost, making it hard to control weight in the future.

There are a few things we can do that help with a fairly rapid summer shape up plan...

**Waist slenderizer:** going on a fruit, vegetable and low sodium diet for 7-10 days is a fast way to slenderize your waistline and decrease water retention. You can include other foods that are very high in fiber. This is a super way to clean 5-12+ pounds out your digestive tract/colon while detoxing at the same time. People that eat a conventional American diet can oft times have 5-15 pounds of waste stuck in crevices throughout their colon. If you do a detox, be sure to drink lots of water to help flush toxins out of your system.

There are system cleanse kits available that are really good, my favorite is the Lee Haney 7 Day System Cleanse, it's a 3-way system detox for colon, liver, and kidneys.

**Drink lots of cold water:** when we drink cold water, it has a thermogenic/fat burning effect in that our body has to use calories (units of heat) to warm this water to body temperature and since water has ZERO CALORIES this causes a negative calorie effect.

**Fat burner selection:** there are constantly new fat burners hitting the market and some work really well, and will help increase thermogenic (fat burning) activity along with appetite control. Make sure it comes from a company with a good reputation that has a history of developing good products.

**Fat burner usage:** if you decide to use a fat burner that helps control your appetite, pull back on the usage at least twice a week so you can meet your body's food cravings. Your UP CALORIE days are what help you maintain muscle mass and helps to continue to trick your body into releasing body fat as energy on the low calorie days.

**On your up-calorie days:** you should get a minimum of your body weight x 12 calories, (especially if you're a very active person). Up-calorie days should be on workout days or days when you are most active.

 **Fat-burning exercise routine:** rotating from a pulling exercise, to a pushing exercise, to a leg exercise allows you to work in a continuous circuit, without having to rest since they're different muscle groups. Keeping your heart rate up and working large muscle groups turns your muscle toning routine into a fat burning one as well. You can also do body weight movements that use a lot of muscles throughout the body and by simply increasing the pace, it increases the resistance a lot like adding resistance on an exercise machine.

 We should never force our body to rewind in one month, what we let happen for the last eleven!

Rapid weight loss causes us to lose shape as well as ages our vital organs...

# Getting Our Skin In Shape
# For Summer

Skin is our body's largest organ and is also our last line of defense against our external environment. And just like a gradual conditioning of our skeletal muscle to become capable to handle a heavier workload, our skin requires much the same gradual approach to sun exposure.

We have a big cosmetics industry that benefits if billions of people on earth think that the sun is dangerous, and feel they need their lotions to protect us from it. There are some facts however that they cannot dispute and seem to avoid bringing up when fear mongering the public about the sun:

**Fact:** the sun has been around for 1000's of years.

**Fact:** pretty much everything on planet earth would die without it.

**Fact:** one of the body's main sources of vitamin D is the sun which in turn helps protect us from cancer.

**Fact:** almost all chronic diseases are linked to vitamin D deficiencies.

**Fact:** the deadliest form of skin cancer, melanoma, has been on the rise by about 3.5 percent per year since 1992, according to the American Melanoma Foundation. Interestingly enough, this rise in melanoma has been paralleled by a 4.2 percent increase in sunscreen use...

We can set an environment through our diet and exposure to the sun that helps us condition and rejuvenate our skin, but if we instead choose to slather on sunblock's that are loaded with chemicals and have radical exposure to the sun and or tanning beds, we leave our skin vulnerable to premature aging, wrinkling, and even worse, cancers.

When we work our muscles too hard, we get extremely sore and if we don't back off, we can have cascading joint, tendon and ligament issues that in turn can lead to inflammatory conditions resulting in chronic skeletal conditions.

Our skin is much the same, in that when we over expose our skin to the sun or tanning beds, it can cause an inflammatory condition (fever under the skin), and if this kind of exposure is continued or happens often enough may result in a chronic disease of the skin, such as skin cancer. So the key is in a gradual increase in exposure, prior to long periods of exposure, (like an athlete that builds up strength and endurance leading up to a sporting event).

We all dislike getting burned on the first day of vacation and having the entire trip messed up due to unconditioned skin, that went from an occasional hour a day in the sun to 5 hours. If a beginner did that same thing in a gym he/she would probably be crippled for a few days and if continued could potentially cause permanent damage to the muscle and skeletal function of the body!

**Skin Fitness Tips...**

**1. Lotions:** a highly recommended one is raw Shea

Butter and when necessary use a mineral based sunblock that contains zinc oxide and/or titanium dioxide as the active ingredients. These are safe and they block the sun by sitting on top of our skin, instead of absorbing into our skin. Bottom line, we do not want to slather on endocrine (hormone) disrupting, cancer causing chemicals that we then let the sun bake into our system.

**2. Avoid harsh soaps:** use milder soaps, to avoid stripping the skin of the oils it uses to protect itself. Vitamin D is produced by a chemical reaction between the sun's rays and these oils. This healthy level of vitamin D then helps with cell replication and helps us avoid the same turning into cancerous mutations.

**3. Clothing and other protective gear:** always have light full length clothing, hats etc. that you can put on whenever you feel like your exposure time is too far exceeding the times your skin is used to. Sun umbrellas and shades work great!

**4. Exposure:** just like our immune system and exercising builds strength through consistent exposure, our skin readies itself through exposure.

**5. Diet:** eat your sunscreen, by eating foods that enhance your body's natural defense mechanisms against harmful rays. These foods include (but are not limited to) brightly colored fruits and vegetables, nuts, berries and dark leafy vegetables. These pigments and colors in plant life use the sun to build food, and have their purpose in giving our skin good synergy with the sun.

Our skin is our body's largest organ and is a mirror of what is happening within...

# A Cancerous Lifestyle (?)

Why is it that in the early 1900's only 1 in 30 people were expected to get cancer, but now 1 in 2 men and 1 in 3 women will get cancer in their lifetime? Why is it, after all these years and billions of dollars spent on research, the problem has grown into a giant industry and is a growing problem, not a shrinking one?

Did you know that every 2.5 seconds someone is diagnosed with cancer, every 4 seconds someone dies from cancer? (Quoted from-World Health Organization).

Why are we looking for a cure so much instead of looking for what is causing cancer? Are the ones we're trusting to look for a cure even considering that what we're breathing, consuming, injecting or coming in contact with, just might be the cause of everything they are designing treatments for?

If we know a highway we're traveling on is littered with broken glass and nails, would we choose another route or would we continue on hoping there will be an accessible tire shop and then hope they can make the repair in time so we can still complete the journey we started? Would we expect tire shops and tire companies to cleanup the highways for us so that we could prevent the need for their services? Would it not make more sense to scare people into regularly stopping in to use expensive diagnostic services to check for potential leaks (or pre-leak-leaks) so that they could create a whole new industry of early detection?

Why would drug companies spend research dollars on a cure, when they can develop drugs to MANAGE IT for the balance of the customer's lifespan??? Would it not be a smart move to shape the fear of a disease in a way that people would think the time and $$$ they spend on early detection is more important then the time and effort spent on prevention? Why have we become conditioned to think that early detection is more important then avoiding the things that cause the problem in the first place?

When our body gets sick, it wants to heal itself, why can't we spend time figuring out what it needs to do its job? Our body has an internal physician that works 24 x 7 x 365 building, repairing and defending us and all it asks for is a balanced lifestyle of healthy habits to pull its tools from to build our defenses, is that asking too much?

Do you believe your natural body and systems are designed to respond more favorably to nature, or do you feel the best response comes from toxic chemicals and regular screenings that emit harmful radiation through the body and chemotherapy that literally strips your body of nutrients and its immune system?

Yesterday I was watching an interview on CBS about a very exciting breakthrough on cancer, a study of using ones own immune system to hunt cancer cells (imagine that)" but it was short lived when the news anchor asked him... "Am I hearing CURE" which he rapidly responded that it's not, but instead said that it is something that can manage the cancer and can help someone lead a full life. We should all know that this would only include a full life for continuing customers.

**Ending questions:**

**1.** Did you know that most cancers are the result of chronic inflammation?

**2.** Since inflammation is the source of most chronic disease, including most cancer, why are there not massive amounts of research on acute inflammation becoming chronic inflammation?

**3.** To grow, cancer needs fuel; did you know sugar is fuel to cancer?

# Green Leafy Vegetables
# Look and See Better!

The antioxidants of the eyes are lutein and zeaxanthin. These 2 antioxidants help protect our eyes from oxidative damage that in turn leads to vision loss. Oxidative damage to our body (is like rusting is to a vehicle) and is largely responsible for premature aging and other chronic diseases. Green leafy vegetables (especially the ones dark in color) are loaded with lutein and zeaxanthin! This is the time of year that we have a lot of regionally grown leafy vegetables, as well as the reds, purples, yellows and the whites, so its a great time to get our levels of these nutrients up in our blood to help our body get rid of oxidative damage that may have built up during the winter months.

When we take in nutrients from our food, it basically tells our body what to do, and when we eat a rainbow of different colors in our diet (especially ones grown in our area) we give our body thousands upon thousands of little micronutrients that repair, rebuild and remove toxicities that they are good at getting rid of.

During normal wear and tear our body produces free radicals and these free radicals cause oxidative damage (body rusting). Though they are a part of normal wear and tear, the amount can be increased or decreased by our lifestyle and keeping good levels of antioxidants in our blood helps us combat excessive oxidation. Keeping good levels of lutein and zeaxanthin in our blood supply can help supply our eyes with the tools to clean things up and to help defend themselves against this oxidation.

Our eyes have a lot of exposure and have a really big task in front of them that we oft times take for granted. Our eyes receive information and then transmit it through nerve signaling to our brain, which then elicits a certain response from us whether neutral, negative or positive. Either way we need to hope the transmission continues to work properly or we may see or not see things properly, which will in turn yield a potentially out of whack response.

**Weight loss:** this is the time of year that most of us probably would like to shed a few pounds, which is an added benefit of eating lots of green leafy vegetables, (especially if they're raw or just lightly cooked). Besides upping our metabolism from the increase in the thermic effect (digestion) of these foods, it can also help push out excess colon waste that causes our midsection to be more bloated then it would have to be, (its not always fat that makes the midsection stick out). A good intake of raw vegetables and fruits help to push and drag out toxic waste and residue while slimming our waistline at the same time.

**Top green leafy vegetables:** a favorite of mine is kale, but there are many others such as collard greens, turnip greens, Swiss chard, spinach, mustard greens and though not leafy, broccoli is a part of this lineup.

**Eye exercise:** try putting something small on a ledge or floor such as a marble, then stand a small distance away, and then walk as rapidly as you can past your object and pick it up with your thumb and forefinger without slowing down. If you are able to do this, there is a lot of eye, brain, skeletal, and muscular coordination that just happened!

Having good eyesight is a blessing we should never take for granted and eating for good eye health has the plus side of slimming the waistline as well!

# The Bonus Payout
# From Manual Labor

Physical activity at work (at your paying job) is something I've thought a lot about over the past years, and I see it even more as the warnings continue to come out about sedentary lifestyles, setting still for extended periods, and last but not least, mental stress when not combined with its healthy counterpart which is physical stress.

Inactivity is linked to most chronic disease, (heart disease, cancer, diabetes) and oft times, it's partner in crimes against the body (obesity). If we can counter chronic disease by getting more active, doesn't this include physical work at our job as well?

Whenever I hear of a company that pays their employees for their gym time, I automatically think "smart company" and I can tell it makes the employee feel really good that their company cares about their health and fitness! A company allowing an employee to go to the gym while on the clock, to exercise, improve health, fitness, shape while getting paid, sounds pretty good to most people that care about their health!

However, if we have a physically exhausting job such as carpentry, plumbing, fabrication, waitressing or janitorial, we oft times tend to look at it different then when we exercise in a gym or have paid exercise time from our employer. Its not so different, especially if you can work fast enough to get your heart rate up for an extended period and can go through a variety of movements, such as lifting, pulling, pushing, squatting, and walking.

I really believe with all the environmental toxins, food additives, and stress, when this is combined with a sedentary lifestyle or job, will have a buildup of pending side effects that can really position us at the losing end of the stick, in future healthcare costs, down time, premature aging and chronic disease.

It makes perfect sense that our intake of fast food, processed food, as well as loads of sugar, when combined with lifestyles that are inactive are exactly what is setting this perfect storm for a massive era of death by chronic disease. We can change this by following 3 words, changing lifestyle habits.

There are many health benefits in a job that requires physical output, and this physical activity can have great immediate and long-term benefit.

**Here are a few:** increased muscle mass and tone, increased cardio endurance, better cardiopulmonary circulation, increased bone density, better detoxification and regular bowel movements, physical fatigue from activity or exercise relieves mental stress, lower body fat and last but not least, you get a workout while making money!

**How to get a workout on the job:** when you see a stretch of work that might last 20 minutes or longer, increase the speed that you do it to get your heart rate up, (this helps burn body fat and build cardio endurance). If you want to build muscle density, increase the load or speed of movement.

**If you have a desk job:** stand up and move around whenever you get a chance. You can do some rapid squat thrusts, jumping jacks, or pushups whenever you take a restroom break, (if you take 5-10 breaks, this will add up). If you do an exercise that activates most of your muscles, you can do a lot in one minute of rapid, intense exercise.

When we look at the health benefits of a body that keeps in motion and realize that health will be tomorrow's currency, our appreciation can grow for a job (or daily activities) that keep us on the move and can make us feel like we're accomplishing two things at one time!

After all, its pretty neat if you can work and make a paycheck from your employer while getting exercise at the same time!

"They give you cash which is as good as money"

~ Yogi Berra

# Fat Furnace Trigger

Burning fat is one thing that we have over complicated and commercialized in every feasible way imaginable. Every time we turn around there is a newest, latest best way to burn it for us!

**I have a question:** if we spent a lot of time and money, canning and storing food in our storage pantry, would we pay someone money to come burn some of it, if we felt our inventory had grown too large? Or would we skip going to the grocery store every so often and simply use from our storage supply, thus reducing the size of our inventory?

**How to unlock the door to our storage areas:** many of us probably know that sugar is by far one of the biggest culprits in creating fatty deposits, but just like the creation of fatty deposits the KEY in getting these same fatty deposits to release the calories they store, is in getting the SUGAR in our blood LOW!

**How our body stores fat:** our body produces insulin whenever it senses sugar entering our system, (this is how glucose gets transported to muscle cells for energy). Whenever we take in more sugar then our muscle cells need, the insulin will continue to transport it out of our blood, but this is when it starts stuffing it into our fat cells, making them fat. If insulin were not doing this, our veins, arteries etc. would become a sticky mess causing anything from blindness to loss of circulation leading to amputations!

**Fat Burning Trigger:** since sugary intake (especially lots of sugar and starches) causes our pancreas to release insulin to do it's job, oft times once the sugar is transported, (if we don't continue to fuel this fire with more sugar) we will feel our energy start to bottom out. The reason is simple, we flooded our system with too many little workers (insulin) and they depleted our sugar!

This is when we oft times make the mistake of thinking we need to take in some sugar, DON'T!!! Just drink some really cold water and try to move around for a while and this will help speed up and trigger the next reaction. Once all the insulin in our blood figures out the sugar is gone, our level of insulin will recede from our blood and this is the trigger that actually opens the door to receiving energy into our system from the fat cells. So its actually 2 things that need to get low, before our body starts to get it's energy from stored fat, sugar then insulin.

Two of the worse things in the obesity epidemic are beverages that are not water and sweet foods without fiber! A sweet food or drink without fiber to slow down sugar's entry into our bloodstream, when consumed will effectively shut down the burning of body fat for energy!

Why has our era of FDA and USDA controlled food and drug system along with new diet foods, weight loss bars, weight loss drinks, fat burners, and other easy weight loss methods yielded an explosive era of obesity and chronic disease?

I believe the answer is a simple one; we have entered an era where we have lazily let people (we have no business trusting), do our thinking for us and they have gotten us off track as to what the basic fundamentals of weight loss and disease prevention actually are!

**Free weight loss plan:** figure out how much fat you want to burn off, then select the days you are least active and not exercising to eliminated starches and sugars (this includes fruits). Doing intermittent fasting on your non-exercise days). Drink half your body weight in ounces of water, (drinking cold water between meals helps burn more calories).

With the cost of food, and the time that it takes for us to eat it, there is no reason that weight loss should not save us time and money.

# Pain Pills are Blinders of Fact

When we put on a set of blinders so that we can no longer see something, it does not change the fact that it's still there. And the fact that we cannot see what is developing right in front of us because we purposely keep a set of blinders on could do us a lot of harm if we do not have proper function to react to things that are happening around us!

We have gone down a path of least resistance by accepting hook line and sinker (as a society) what we should do about symptoms of underlying problems that cause us pain. When we cannot feel the pain and continue to do the things that cause our body to hurt, would it not make the problem get worse?

**Example:** a knee that is hurting due to elements in the joint grinding together... What would feel best to the knee, to be supported with a knee brace and strengthening the muscles around it to better support weight and function, or regularly taking pain medicine so we cannot feel what it's going through? Pain medicine has its place, but not without an action plan on what needs to be done to get off!

This growth is spurred by an industry that benefits from treating symptoms of pain on a continual basis instead of finding and drying out the root cause of the pain. This same industry would lose out big time, if people immediately after starting pain medicine, would enact an exit strategy to get off.

If we followed the money trail and would see the massive amount of profits that are made from the prescription narcotics drug industry, (from drug addiction) we would have a better understanding why we are not allowed to raise our own free herbal pain medicine. However, when something is in fact addictive, mind altering, harmful to organs of the body, turns many people into society damaging pain pill junkies, financially ruining many people's lives as well as that of their families and has caused more death then cocaine and heroin combined, we somehow think continued use is okay because we have a prescription. This way of thinking is not a whole lot different then that of a preprogramed robot!

Many of these pain medicines give someone a feeling of euphoria and will cause actual physical pain when you try to get off them, and whether they are formulated this way or not, it certainly keeps a growing repeat customer base for the pharmaceutical companies that are in the pain pill industry.

We have got to get back to thinking for ourselves instead of letting ones (that profit from our actions, inaction, and decisions), do our thinking for us. After all its your liver, not theirs!

Most chronic pain come from chronic inflammatory conditions, and this continued inflammatory condition is being caused by something that is being aggravated. We don't just need to take a pain medicine, and we don't just need to just take a anti-inflammatory medicine, we need to FIND OUT what is aggravating our body. Aggravation left unattended will eventually produce a diseased condition in the area of chronic inflammation.

**Questions:** if chronic disease (whether bone, muscle or organ) is painful to the body, but we continue to take pain medicine, does it not put us out of touch with finding the source of our dis-ease and discomfort? If we are regularly taking addictive pain medicine without finding and getting rid of what is causing the pain, does that not make us a drug addict, whether with or without a prescription? The liver is involved in over 500 functions throughout the body, should we continue taking anything that has a negative affect on the liver?

### Tracking chronic pain:

**1.** Find source of pain

**2.** Find source of inflammation

**3.** Find cause of aggravation, (taking care of aggravation, cools and dries out inflammation, which in turn eliminates pain).

To continue using pain medicine to deal with pain or for doctors to continue prescribing them to patients (without an exit strategy) is akin to giving someone a bucket for a leaky boat instead of finding and fixing the leak.

# Health and Fitness Fundamentals

**Definition of fundamental-** basic: relating to or affecting the underlying principles or structure of something.

One of my all time favorite quotes is, "Ask why, and ask it again five more times, until all the artifice is stripped away and you end up with the intellectually honest answer." ~ Andy Grove

If we know what the fundamental (the root) is for a subject matter, we should be able to better question principles people try to put in place that claim to "fix it, repair it, remedy it, enhance or even better it."

We have somehow allowed the market, society, government, greed and laziness to come in and give us a twisted perception of health, wealth, freedom and happiness. When we get off track from the underlying fundamentals on any of the above, and it is not stopped, we can expect an erosive affect whether it be personally or that of a society.

The fundamentals of health really do not change, and if we can learn what these basics are, (the simple things our body likes) we can pretty easily track backwards to find out where a health problem, obesity problem, mobility problem etc. stems from.

**Example:** obesity doesn't come from not having a membership to a health club, from not taking weight loss drugs or fat burners nor does it come from not having home exercise equipment. Obesity comes from eating too much in comparison to a person's level of activity and muscle, its simple as that, nothing more and nothing less. When we address our level of activity, our amount of muscle and muscle tone as well as calorie intake, we address obesity.

When we know what actually caused the problem (obesity) in the first place, all that is left is how we can best address the three things that caused it, which is to decrease calorie intake and increase physical activity that in turn builds or tones muscle and helps burn off excess calories.

There are some basic fundamentals to good health and most things that go wrong with our health can be traced backwards to one or more of these. When we bring these back into balance, our health will begin to do the same.

**Basic fundamentals:**

**1.** Clean Air.

**2.** Water.

**3.** Balanced diet.

**4.** Sunshine.

**5.** Exercise/Activity.

**6.** Sleep.

What each one of the above do for our health is very important and when lacking in either of the above can lead us down the path of, cancer, heart disease, diabetes, mobility issues, lack of energy, obesity, arthritis, constipation, bad physical appearance, rapid aging and the list goes on and on! Many of these are only symptoms of an underlying problem and are not the root problem AT ALL!!!

Whenever we are experiencing any of the above symptoms, we should immediately look for what factors can cause that symptom, then simply check it against our checklist of healthy fundamentals and see if we fall short on any.

**Example:** if we're chronically tired, we can go through the checklist and if we sleep good, get plenty clean air, have a balanced diet, get plenty of sunshine, and stay active, but we don't drink water like we should, (lack of hydration is probably the problem) and very likely we're having millions of cells dying each day due to a lack of hydration, which in turn could be the root cause of the chronic fatigue.

### 6 Questions we should ask:

**1.** What is my problem?

**2.** What is causing it?

**3.** Could the solution I'm being offered cause more problems eventually then I'm having now?

**4.** Is this to help manage a symptom, or is it a cure for the problem?

**5.** What can I do personally to change it?

**6.** Am I worth doing it the right way?

Health fundamentals are basic and very simple to understand. If they become confusing or hard to understand, it's probably for someone else's benefit and not that of your own...

# Stay Hydrated, or You'll Start Shutting Down!!!

Our body has a really awesome cooling system, but it quickly loses its effectiveness when fluid and electrolyte levels get low or depleted! This dehydration can lead to heat exhaustion and stroke due to not having the fluid levels in our body to properly expel the heat.

This time of the year, one of the most important things to keep in mind when spending time outside, is to stay hydrated with cold water and an occasional cold electrolyte/sports drink.

**Dehydration and how it works:** our body will kick off a process called arginine vasopressin which will cause a reaction from our kidneys to begin concentrating its elimination of urine to conserve fluid in the body. As we become further dehydrated our body will completely shut down the elimination of fluids leaving the body (by shutting down the kidneys)! As these survival mechanisms kick in we can expect other functions to slow down or quit working in favor of more important functions.

The above situation can rapidly deteriorate when there is a high level of physical activity, ambient (surrounding) heat or a combination of both!

The most vital supplement to life is oxygen, and our blood needs enough volume (plasma) to carry and deliver oxygen rich blood cells throughout our body. Even though other things may start drying out and shutting down, when our oxygen delivery system starts failing due to lack of hydration, we can pretty much expect that we're about to check out of this life!

I just recently experienced a little of the same, when I was outside working for around 5 hours, I simply did not pay as much attention as I should've, to stay hydrated and noticed later that I never had to urinate the entire time, but when I got home it was very concentrated.

As a general rule, we want to try to drink around half our bodyweight in ounces of water, and this needs to be adjusted upward, depending how much activity or heat our body and its systems are exposed to.

**Example:** a 150-pound person would drink 75 ounces of water.

Staying properly hydrated doesn't mean simply drinking massive amounts of water, since this can gradually wash out our electrolytes, which in turn will cause our body to not properly retain fluids. Btw sodium isn't a bad thing, it helps hold fluids in suspension evenly throughout our body and keeps it from dropping down around our ankles!

Sport drinks and homemade electrolyte drinks are designed to replenish these electrolytes.

**Sweating and gas vapor:** our body expels heat by sweating and emitting moisture in the form of gas vapor from the skin and both methods use water.

**Diet:** there can also be dietary factors that can cause us to dehydrate more rapidly such as a low glycemic/carb diet. You can help offset this by having a carb increase every 3-4 days.

**Sodium:** if our sodium level gets too low, we inhibit the body's capability to retain fluid. We should make sure we get at least 1400-2000 milligrams of sodium per day (increasing or decreasing) depending on our size, and then increase or decrease according to our activity and heat exposure.
**Note:** most people do not have to worry about sodium levels if they regularly eat out, since most menu items have an overload of sodium.

**Things to watch for:** sharp decrease in sweating and urination, a clammy or dry mouth, and an increase in heart rate due to less blood plasma volume.

**Tips:** when increasing internal heat through activity or being exposed to external heat, drink several rounds of water then switch up to an electrolyte/sports drink. All fluids should be cold, to assist the body in its job of cooling.

If you help your body's cooling system along with proper hydration, it will not put such a drain on your body's energy bill and will protect your body from excessive wear and tear!

# Food, Activity and Sleep Journals

Most anyone that knows me knows that I believe food is our best source of medicine. We have gotten off track in too quickly turning to medicines that attempt to mimic the effects of food. When we find the foods that are good for certain things, (and lean our diet more heavily in that direction) we give our body an anecdote without the side effects of pharmaceutical medicine. It's the difference in medicine from a Farmacy vs. a Pharmacy!

A very powerful health tool is to simply keep track of your food, fluid, activity and sleep habits for 10-15 days. It's a good way to find out what makes your engine run smoothly, efficiently and energetically!

Most whole foods, (vegetables, fruits, nuts, beans, berries, fermented foods, eggs, raw milk, meats from good origin, as well as most food products that are in their original whole food form), have powerful individual medicinal effects. Some give us energy, some give us nutrients that build our blood, some help replenish enzymes in our digestive tract, some help rebuild broken down muscle fibers, some help clean out our digestive tract, some help calm the body from stress, and some help fight inflammation and disease!

There are some foods that do not work well for certain people and yield what we know as food allergies. Just like medicine this could be a reaction to any amount of the food, or getting too much of a certain food. Food allergies can cause acute reactions or ones that are subtler, such as fatigue, headaches etc. These foods need to be tracked down and either reduced or eliminated from your diet.

We need proteins, fats, carbs and the thousands of micronutrients (vitamins, minerals etc.) that are in whole foods. Many of the small nutrients are still unnamed, and we may not know why they're there, but the plant does, and our body certainly does, (imagine an internal pharmacist that has 10's of thousands of specific designer medicines to select from based on your individual needs)!

**If we keep the simple basics in mind when it comes to our diet,** (proteins, fats, carbs, along with vitamin and mineral rich vegetables, fruits, nuts, beans and enzyme rich foods), it becomes much easier to keep a running ledger in our brain of what we have been getting too much or not enough of.

**Example:** If you have a turkey sandwich for lunch, you have protein and fat from the turkey and cheese and carbs from the bread). If you eat nutrient rich fruit(s) or vegetable(s) along with it, it's a fairly balanced meal. If you feel you need to add extra nutrients from these different groups, such as protein and micronutrients, you can add amino acids, multi-vitamin/mineral, or fruit and vegetable extracts to help supplement your meal.

**Food and habit journals:** this is a good way to track a problem down. Simply write down your food and fluid intake as well as your activities and sleep schedules for about 10-15 days. Each day write out the side of the page how you felt periodically throughout the day and evening. After about 10-15 days you should be able to see the days that you felt good, with lots of energy and vitality as well as the foods you ate prior to that time period. Feeling good is the best indicator that you're supplying your body with the right things to get or keep you healthy.

**Foods for healing:** we can use the internet to search for foods that help with most problems, whether it's the best diet for cancer, heart disease, stroke prevention, energy, sleep, diabetes, gastrointestinal issues, gout, vision loss etc. When we get a list of foods (that we like) that match up with our health concern, we can simply add these into our diet and as we do this, we'll find that we push out the ones that are potentially causing our body discomfort and dis-ease.

If we ask ourselves simple basic questions about our diet, our activities, and sleep habits, our research will yield a good prescription for ourselves, or someone we care about.

Many of us know exactly what the basic needs are for our vehicle and will check these things before taking it to a shop to get diagnostics run on it, but will not learn the simple basics that make our body run smoothly and will quickly turn to invasive diagnostic procedures and chemicals for health and prevention.

# Fat Burners That Are Cheap and Free

Most of us either have a few fat pounds we would like to get rid of, but are faced with a confusingly huge selection of fat burners and weight loss plans.

First look at your body's fat as something you spent time, effort and money building, (this is your body's reserve food pantry). So if we do it the right way, (we can save money on food and save time eating it as well) if we begin utilizing and burning our stored calories.

**Fat release trigger:** lowering blood sugar is one of the best ways to trigger the release of body fat so that we can burn it as energy. You can do this by, eliminating sugar and starches for a few days or doing a complete fast for 18-24 hours.

**Cheap thermogenic:** coffee and an aspirin work really well at stimulating thermogenic (fat burning) activity throughout a workout or sporting event. You get stimulated internal heat from the coffee and caffeine as well as an increased blood flow from the aspirin, (stay well hydrated, as it does have diuretic properties).

**Cold Water between meals:** drinking really cold water between meals helps boost thermogenic activity due to the release of calories to warm the water up to regular body temperature, (calories are units of heat/energy). This also works when the body is in a cold external environment, it will release calories (units of heat) to help maintain our body temperature at approximately 98.6 degrees. Whether it's cold or heat, our body burns a lot of calories, maintaining body temperature.

**Note:** cold water or fluid during a meal is counter productive due to our body trying to send warm blood and other digestive juices to our stomach area during and right after a meal.

**Exercise or physical activity as a fat burner:** to turn your workout or physical activity into a fat burning session, simply keep your heart rate at about 120-140 beats per minute, (increase or decrease according to age). After about 20 minutes, it triggers the release of body fat for energy, (many of us know this as our 2nd wind).

Though there are some very good fat burner products and weight loss systems available on the market, you should never feel you have to spend money to lose weight.

Losing weight can save you time and money, simply by triggering your body's mechanism that help us use what we already have in our storage areas.

# Fat, Sick, Tired and Broke

There are things that can suppress the health and economy of people and it is linked directly to a suppression of knowledge, confusion, fear, and simply deferring people's attention away from basic fundamentals.

I believe the above has been made easier by society's increased faith in man and a decreased faith in our Maker which in turn has cause us to drift away from the basics and opt instead for things with flare and a great sounding verbal spin...

We slow down our levels of activity without slowing down our fuel intake, and then complain about weight gain.

We artificially stimulate our metabolism with diet pills and other stimulants instead of losing weight through proper diet, exercise and rebuilding our metabolism through, toning, strengthening and building muscle.

We take pain pills to ignore pain, and then wonder why the origin of the pain doesn't get better or simply gets worse.

We prosecute people for raising a natural herbal painkiller that could be raised for free, but think continuous prescriptions for addictive, (narcotic level) pain pills are okay, (that turn many people into a much more destitute form of a drug addict).

We have an FDA that okays the usage of such chemicals in bread that are used in tennis shoes and yoga mats, but try to convince our politicians and the public that raw milk is hazardous to our health. Milk has been around for 1000's of years and production standards have increased, not decreased!

We take antidepressants to ignore problems, and then wonder why we need them even more at a later date.

We take arthritis drugs but do not bother to strengthen muscles that will help lift and support our body's weight to relieve the bones and joints from (inflammation causing) weight sagging on our bones, causing arthritic conditions.

We take lots of antibiotics and take in far fewer probiotics or probiotic rich foods to replace the probiotics (that the antibiotics have killed) and then wonder why our gastric tract gives us anti-digestive problems.

We clog up the most important ingredient for life (oxygen) with cigarette smoke and other chemicals.

We clog up the 2nd most important ingredient to life (water) with colorings, caffeinating, sugars and carbonation.

We sanitize our surroundings with toxic chemicals to kill germs, but create a cancerous environment in the process.

We have a cancer/tumor industry that tries to convince us that we need immediate invasive, poisonous procedures and then continuous medicine, and checkups rather then aligning the patient with a nutritionist and a anti-cancerous lifestyle. Everyone that is not yet diagnosed with cancer already fights cancer everyday, EVERYONE including you and I!

We eat lots of goo that sticks to our intestinal walls with very few raw vegetables in-between to break it up and move it along and then wonder why we are so constipated.

We guzzle liquid, carbonated, caffeinated, sugar loaded drinks and mass-produce sweet foods without (soluble fiber in them to slow down sugar absorption), and then wonder why our pancreas gets worn out and why we have a diabetes epidemic.

We opt to get on a lifetime supply of diabetes medicine to command our body to bloat our fat cells with these continued surges of sugar, instead of changing what we eat.

We weaken our immune system by sanitizing our surroundings and try to live in a sanitized bubble, but then inject simulated funk (vaccinations) that only guesses at our future germ exposures.

We have adapted to a source of food that is largely made from processed sources and brought in from various parts of the country instead of, from plant life that uses the energy from sun, wind, rain and soil from the region we live in.

Last but not least, health and financial issues are probably the cause of most of the stress in our adult lives, so why isn't more time spent in the last year of grade school, dedicated simply on avoiding the pit falls of these two?

Education benefits the masses, however the profits (from debt, disease, fear and suppression of energy efficiencies) massively benefit a select few.

# Supporting Our Roadside Farmers Markets

This is a business that is growing in popularity and I really hope it continues to grow! If you're in this business, your business should continue to grow over the coming years, especially if you have good grower connections and public access spots. It would be great if eggs from free range chickens and raw pet milk (punt intended) were included in your services as well.

Over the years we have developed logistics that can rapidly move foods from one region to another and it has probably gotten us a little off track as to what foods we really should be eating. This combined with grower associations that target their marketing in regions and countries that they want to market their products to. This can make us feel like we are picking a superior food, when we choose something over a locally grown food.

**Georgia example:** thinking the walnut (California) is better then the pecan, the orange (Florida) is nutritionally better then a peach, cashews (Brazil) better then peanuts, noni or goji berries (Hawaii and China) are better then blue or blackberries.

**Vine ripened:** vine or plant ripened produce is nutritionally better then ones picked prior to ripening. I like to think of vine ripened as being the point at which the plant is fully ready to release the project it has been working on and perfecting for a long time. Have you noticed how hard it is to get a plant to release it's product when its not ripe, but how easily it releases it once it's finished?

When produce is picked and shipped from another part of the country to another, it is almost impossible to pick at the ripened stage due to spoilage.

I have a friend that moved to England and fell in love with the way they bring local grown produce,

151

eggs and milk to market, which is their doorstep! Hopefully there will be more individuals setting up routes through neighborhoods, business districts etc. in the future to broker high quality local grown produce and dairy products from producer to consumer. We have technology that can help with speed of order delivery, mobile payments and customer tracking, so the capability for growth of the farm to market business should be really good!

Not only is this a good thing nutritionally for the people in an area and region, but an economical one as well. If this becomes a more viable cash business for the farmer, we will have more growers taking part and when there is more competition, quality of goods and services tends to go up.

If we can find out where the roadside stands and farmers markets are around us, and every so often, stop in and buy a few things, we can help this become a better business for them and make it worth their time to continue their business in our area the next year.

Most naturally grown foods, spices, herbs etc. have nutritional and medicinal qualities wherever their place of origin is, but...

Foods grown in another region simply do not have the overall medicinal capabilities (designed for you) that foods have, that are grown in your area.

# Vertical Stimulation...Avoiding Excess Fluid Retention

If we are fairly active, we do this without thinking about it. Rapid vertical movement stimulates our lymphatic system and increases its circulation.

Our lymphatic system is sort of a catchall and plays a large role in our immune system's proper function. If the lymph fluid does not get circulated, it can cause swelling, stagnation of the lymph fluid, subsequent illness and cancer formation. This fluid has to be pushed up through the lymph nodes for cleaning, and then disposal. It does this through surrounding muscle contractions.

There are lots of fluids that empty into and then are transported through our lymph system, so it works really well at rapidly detecting bad things entering the body. Our lymph nodes (that are placed throughout the lymphatic system) are like substations that everything has to pass through and when they detect a disease or infection, they will release a flood of white blood cells into our system to fight and eliminate whatever this foreign invader is.

Our lymph nodes are positioned all over our body like little police stations and all this fluid has got to pass through them to be inspected as well as neutralizing the bad things when they come through. There are around 1,000 nodes placed very strategically around our body. Our abdomen has around 300, so it can rapidly detect bad things in our food and can quickly alert our immune system.

There are two things that happen, our nodes not only kill the pathogen and then transport it out through one of our waste systems, it will also send out white blood cells (lymphocytes) to track down and kill the source of the infection or disease. The increase in white blood cells is how a doctor detects the presence of an infection or disease.

**Vertical stimulation:** up and down motion is the way our lymph fluid moves upwards toward filtration and then out through one of our debris (trash) removal systems. Our lymph vessels have valves that are aimed in the direction the flow is supposed to go, to prevent back flow, then once it gets to the end of the thoracic duct our excess fluids and its waste products get sent for removal through our feces, urine, lungs and skin. Exercise helps this fluid move and helps us with fluid retention problems, through increased elimination.

Some of the best ways to stimulate the lymph system is on a trampoline or rebounder (small trampoline), however most exercises especially ones that have rapid vertical movements, (jumping jacks etc.) should help keep this system active, healthy and keep fluid from building up in areas and turning rancid.

The above is very important to do and with regularity. Unlike our blood, which has a heart to pump and circulate it, our lymph system depends on activity for its circulation.

If you have a health crisis such as cancer, systemic infections etc., you really should get a rebounder trampoline to stimulate the immune system and to help it remove the bad stuff. Strengthening and assisting the immune system is a really good place to start your fight to regain health.

Our lymphatic system is like a giant fluid supply system, cleansing system for our cells, processing system for dead cells, filtration system, drainage system, as well as an alert system with its own immune system military! All it asks from us is MOVEMENT!!!

# Gastric Trouble Makers...Healing Our Gut

We have a digestive tract that has a massive duty of processing our food and helping us extract nutrients we need to keep our body energized, and fed with nutrients that help us fight disease and aging. Unfortunately something that gets overused and abused will gradually get tired, aged and less capable to do its job.

One of the biggest culprits is dead food that has been frozen, overcooked, baked, grilled or fried. These foods still supply us with very vital macronutrients, fat, protein, and carbs), but do not supply us with live enzymes, so our body has to use of its own supply to breakdown and process these foods with an inadequate amount of replacement enzymes coming in. As these enzymes get depleted, our digestive tract simply has fewer workers to help us break down the food we eat.

Chewing our food properly helps save gut energy, (by beginning the breakdown process of the food as well as mixing in the enzymes that are supposed to be added in, prior to sending it to the stomach). Our digestion is a step-by-step process and if not finished properly in our mouth, our stomach has to make up for it.

**Foods that do not decompose rapidly:** have you ever noticed how long a processed snack food lasts before it decomposes? When a food does not have the enzymes that decomposes itself, our digestive tract has got to do all the work, but when foods are loaded with enzymes it brings little workers into our digestive tract that help replenish the digestive work force. Our modern food logistic systems hate enzyme rich foods, because these foods do not last as long. So killing the enzyme activity by radiation, especially in fruits and vegetables are in their best interest, (especially super market and restaurant chain produce). They still have nutrient quality, just much less then vine ripened, non-radiated local grown produce.

**Leaky gut:** most anytime our body gets aggravated in an area, it will get puffy and inflamed. This is simply our body's natural immune response, but when it continues and developed into chronic inflammation, (if not stopped) will develop into a chronic disease. This can happen to our digestive tract as well and cause the cells lining our digestive tract to have more space between them, which allows food particles that are not properly digested to pass through and get into our bloodstream. This inflammation can be caused by anything that aggravates our digestive tract, whether continued use of antibiotics, infections, food allergies to things such as gluten etc. Most autoimmune diseases come from food particles entering the blood, thus triggering the body to produce antibodies that cause systemic inflammation throughout our body. When this continues to happen long enough, we are apt to produce diagnosable symptoms such as lupus, fibromyalgia, multiple sclerosis, Crohn's disease, chronic fatigue, rheumatoid arthritis and many others.

**Avoiding leaky gut:** keep track of anything that upsets your stomach. If you have to take antibiotics, make sure you counter its effects with probiotics. Ask your doctor when you should take the antibiotic and when you should take the probiotic.
**Note:** probiotics and antibiotics can get really ticked if taken together, (they are very much opposite)! Antibiotics kill life in the gut, (both good and bad), probiotics increase life in the gut, so when these are taken together, they go to war with each other.

**Gallbladder removal:** our gallbladder stores bile from our liver to help us break down fat in our diet. If you have had your gallbladder removed, you probably have digestive issues whenever you eat a high fat meal, and you should probably use bile salt tablets. Other supplements that may help are Choline and Betaine. You can purchase them at most vitamin/supplement shops.

**Gut medicine:** you can begin healing your digestive tract and replenish your enzyme supply by eating fresh, raw, vine ripened, locally grown fruits and vegetables. You can rebuild a healthy digestive gut flora plus your capability to fight belly fat by adding in onions, artichokes, asparagus, avocado, leafy greens, garlic, kiwi, water with lemon, apple cider, probiotic rich yogurt and Sauerkraut. I highly recommend taking an enzyme supplement, especially if you already have digestive issues. Most supplement stores have these available, (ask for the best quality).

**Tips:** don't drink a lot of cold fluid during meals, this is very counterproductive to the digestive process when we dump a lot of cold fluid into our stomach right when it's trying to heat up this area for digestion. If you have digestive issues, keep a simple food and fluid journal to log your food intake, fluid intake and to write in periodically how you feel. Our intake is supposed to energize and help us feel good, not bad!

Over 2,000 years ago, Hippocrates said "all disease begins in the gut," so lets do as he says in his most famous quote..."Let thy food be thy medicine and medicine be thy food"~ Hippocrates

# The Power of the Cherry!

An article about cherries recently caught my attention and I thought it really interesting that cherries were ranked #1 in the list of powerful anti-inflammatory foods.

Inflammation is usually at the root of pain and when inflammation continues in an area, it becomes what we know as chronic inflammation, and is what usually leads to chronic disease.

**For joint pain:** cherries have long been known to help with gout and osteoarthritis, and studies have shown that the anthocyanins and phenolics in tart cherries have a powerful effect in reducing inflammation that can cause joint pain, (which if left festering can lead to degenerative joint conditions).

**Arthritis:** osteoarthritis is the most common type of arthritic conditions and is known as "wear and tear" arthritis, (which many people have to deal with as they get older) and can especially be prevalent in athletes or other lifestyles in which the joints catch a lot of impact which can lead to wear and tear, eventually yielding an arthritic condition of the joints. During times of high levels of physical stress, an intake of tart cherries or tart cherry juice, may help ward off the inflammatory conditions and pain you might otherwise have.

**Muscle pain:** long distance runners that use tart cherry juice during their training, have been shown to have less muscle pain after a long distance run, then ones who trained without it. I believe this could possibly be a good bet for other muscle aches and maladies as well, (its not like you have to worry about the potential side effects of a pharmaceutical medicine misdiagnosis).

Since inflammation is an immune response to aggravation and injury, we should remember that we should always to go back one step further and figure out what is causing the inflammation. If we take an anti-inflammatory to shrink the inflammation without addressing whatever is aggravating the body's immune system, we are working against ourselves! Not dealing with what is causing the inflammation is like trying to dry a floor but forgetting to turn off the spigot where the water is coming from in the first place.

**Example:** if our knee, ankle, elbow, neck, back etc. is bothering us, brace it up or put a support around it so that it can heal. A band or brace helps protect and support a vulnerable area much like body armor; it helps deflect things that come at you that could otherwise injure you.

**Power compounds in cherries:** the antioxidant compounds in cherries (anthocyanins) not only give it that bright red color, it also has been linked to high antioxidant capacity and reduced inflammation at levels comparable to some well-known pain medications.

Isn't it neat that a bright red color from nature's Farmacy can help us get rid of red puffy inflammation in the body, without the list of side effects that pain medicine and anti-inflammatory drugs may have!

# Researching For Cures Instead of Causes

The research for cures is usually deeply funded, because of the monetary value of a new medicine that will be developed for this condition. Have you noticed how many of these medicines once developed are for managing the disease and not at all for curing it?

Most of the funding from these BIG movements to raise public awareness transfers massive amounts of money from the public to the pharmaceutical research industry (while at the same time stimulating fear of the disease and then the following subjection to the medicine once a matching medicine is formulated). Oft times the same people that scare people then offer a solution...

Disease and its origins are a very valuable resource for generating billions of dollars for big pharmaceutical companies and their shareholders. For us to think their research (or the associations that are gathering funding from the public for the pharmaceutical industry) is for squashing the ugly origin of the disease, is simply not looking at how much it benefits them to keep the disease alive and well.

**Example:** the American Cancer Society was founded by John D. Rockefeller Sr. in 1913 (after having founded the Rockefeller Institute for Medical Research in 1901) along with some prominent business leaders and physicians at the Harvard Club in New York. Although funding for cancer research and awareness has been massive since then, cancer has exploded into the number 2 leading killer of Americans. Maybe the American Cancer Society's twin snakes and sword symbol is symbolic of something other then healing medicine and diagnostics. This same education system formed in the early 1900's has since then made the advocates of natural remedies out to be quacks.

**Confusing labels:** whenever a new symptom is discovered (or a new disorder named), it then has a strong possibility that a new medicine can be developed to manage it, and if there are a lot of people that can be diagnosed with this disorder or disease the better it is, this means a huge customer base for the developer of the new drug. Confusion and fear, followed by a smart sounding solution often creates a willing patient/consumer.

**Example:** in the U.S. Standard reference for psychiatry (DSM-lV) there are over 300 different manifestations of mental illness. One of these is Conduct Disorder...really!? Didn't we call that misbehavior longer ago, with a good ole butt whooping prescribed as best medicine!?

Even though, most chronic disorders originate from a person's lifestyle habits, more attention is put into which medicine is best for managing the ongoing symptoms, rather then addressing the origin!

**In the early 1900's:** the Rockefeller Foundation helped shape modern medicine (through academic literature, and research funding) and helped move it away from traditional medicine, and though John D. Rockefeller was one of the main advocates of newly formed drugs, he refused personal usage of them and opted for the usage of traditional holistic medicines for his own health.

Medical university funding is largely made possible by the pharmaceutical industry, either directly or indirectly, so what do you think would happen to a university that required its medical students to study the effects of nutrition on the body as well as other healthy lifestyle habits?

If the money, time and efforts spent on trying to find a cure, would be spent instead, on educating the public on the origin of the disease, the reasons for trying to find a cure for it would wither away. But as they say... "He who pays the piper calls the tune."

# Kids and Trapped Classroom Pathogens

This is something that happens to students of all ages, (whether grade school or college) and when being confined day after day together, we can only hope our child's innate immune system (pre-built) is strong enough to ward off the things he or she comes in contact with.

**Innate immune system:** this is the part of the immune system that silently fights and eliminates the bad things we encounter. It does this because of us having encountered it before, and building immunity to it. We do NOT build this part our children's immune system by trying to keep their lives sanitized.

**Acquired immunity:** when they get exposed to germs and other things that could potentially make them sick, their body will not only fight back, it will catalog a memory of this for the next time they encounter a similar bacteria or virus, and without them, or us as parents knowing it, their immune system will basically chop it up, process it, and spit it out! One of my members who had taught school for a few years, said that in the beginning she would come down with almost anything the children brought into the classroom, but after several flu seasons, she could be around almost anything and not worry about being affected! This was her innate immune system learning and sequencing itself into a smart battle machine that had learned almost every strategy the foreign invaders could come up with. Each time our immune system gets exposed it becomes stronger and smarter. If we avoid exposure, (just like an unused muscle), it becomes weak.

**Rest and recovery:** is something that is oft times overlooked until it's too late to avoid a full-blown case of the flu! Getting adequate rest and recovery whenever the immune system encounters something new, is very important in keeping a new virus or bacteria from bringing our child down!

**Watching for signs of exposure:** we need to watch for signs of fatigue for several days after potential exposure, (that's a good sign his or her body is directing its energy to the immune system). When you detect this, your child needs rest, without stimulants such as sugar, caffeine and a lot of surrounding activity!

**Student Nutrition:** a nutritious, balanced diet is very important in building and maintaining a strong immune system! This requires good sources of proteins, fats, vitamins and minerals as well as the many other micronutrients that come from whole food, such as fruits, vegetables and nuts. Increasing intake of foods that are rich in vitamin C, along with extra vitamin C supplementation when eating these foods can help as well. Adding in a good multivitamin can be beneficial as well, however be sure to research the product and company. My preference is fruit and vegetable extract powders, either in capsule form or drink mixes with extra vitamin C and vitamin D supplementation.

**Avoiding stimulants:** besides mental up and downs for a student, this can also wear down a young person's defense mechanisms. If you're a college student, using some coffee to get yourself through an exam or tough period can be okay, (if you allow your body to crash, catch up and recharge). Another downside of stimulants (coffee, and caffeinated beverages) is agitation and brain fog as the stimulant is wearing off, thus leading many to stimulant dependency.

**Activity is the best stimulator of the lymph system,** (which is a huge part of the immune system). Keeping our children's lymph systems moving its fluid along through the lymph nodes, helps kill and get rid of the bad stuff that enters their systems. So active recess times not only relaxes and clears the brain from mental clutter, it can also play a very vital part of keeping his or her immune system healthy!

**Tip:** If your student appears fatigued for no apparent reason, (they may have come in contact with a pathogen that is trying to make them sick), and while their body is working on this, other activities need to be kept minimal, so energy can be redirected to helping the immune system do battle! Also immediately switch to foods that are very easy to digest, so energy normally used in digestion can go to the immune system.

Keeping our child's immune system strong, helps keep them from bringing the flu bugs back home to us, and ain't nobody got time for that!

# Mental and Physical Adversity

There are a lot of parallels that can be drawn between mental stress and physical stress, (and if managed properly, we can become both physically and mentally capable to handle greater and more complex future stresses).

A body and mind left unchallenged will become weak!

**As children:** we can see rapid enhancements in both mental and physical capabilities in a person's first 30 years and then a similar decline of either in the latter 30 years of the normal lifespan.

**Example:** a baby gets really upset the first few times the parents leave, but after it happens a few times, their brain forms connect-a-dots, that tell them it's not the end of life as they knew it to be. This series of connect-a-dots continues to grow, expanding a child's reasoning capabilities throughout his or her childhood, helping them prepare a foundation for continuing academics and learning as a student. The more of these connect-a-dots (reasoning capabilities) we can help our children form outside the classroom, the greater their capability in the classroom. In other words, don't blame the teacher for a job that was and is partly yours. It works the same way in physical capabilities, if we want them to keep up with the other kids on the playground, track or field, we need to do our part and if we don't, do not blame the coach!

**As youth:** we see the same thing happen in rapid succession (throughout childhood until early twenties) in physical development as well as physical capabilities. This is enhanced if kids are active with things that challenge themselves physically and mentally at the same time, (we see this example in the lightning speed and reaction time of many young athletes).

**As adults however;** many of us tend to go with what we know that we can do and gradually get in a comfortable rut that only gets deeper as we get older. As we slow down challenging both our mental and physical capabilities, we gradually see a decline in both physical and cognitive capabilities, and we oft times relate this to aging, when a lot of it comes from us letting our brain and body get sedentary.

 **As seniors:** we see this happen a lot when someone retires and after about 60+ years of a person being scheduled to do things both mentally and physically, retirement can be a major shock to the entirety of a person's physiological functions, (including the brain). Even if we are enjoying life without a schedule, imagine the shock on the body when suddenly after 60 plus years the brain no longer has forward thinking expectations of the body. I believe God gave us a body to accommodate what the brain expects of it! But when mental expectations slow down, it seems physical function slows down accordingly.

 **Mental and physical combinations:** when we combine intense physical activity with mental activity, it can lead to greater cognitive and physical reaction skills. We see this improvement in most people that speed train. When you move through a set of complicated movements faster, (such as an obstacle course) it forces your eyes, brain and body to learn to work together in rapid succession and since each has to respond in coordination with each other, improvements will start showing in both mental and physical capabilities as well as reaction time.

**Balance in training is key:** we have to balance mental and physical adversity with stress free recovery time, or we will become weaker instead of stronger.

**Stress + Rest and Nutrition = Strengthening Process**

Whether it's our brain forming a new connection that gives us a greater understanding of new things we want to learn about, or if we are trying to build our strength, balance, speed, or cardiovascular endurance, it is done through adversity!

# Oil Pressure!!!

Have you ever felt under pressure about which oils and fats are healthy and which ones we should avoid for our families and ourselves? The list is extensive, olive oil, vegetable oil, pecan oil, vegetable oil, coconut oil, macadamia oil, avocado oil, canola oil, corn oil, soybean oil, peanut oil sunflower oil, safflower oil, sunflower oil, butter, lard, margarine, are all choices we get to make when trying to cleanup our diet, and all these choices are enough to drive you nuts right?

**Example:** lard is starting to be considered the great-misunderstood fat. 40% of its fat is saturated fat, and it has 45% monounsaturated fat, which according to this breakdown makes pig fat a fairly healthy fat source. The breakdown of saturated and monounsaturated fats in beef fat is like the fat in olive oil, (which is touted by most health advocates as healthy for the heart).

**Warning:** this is fat straight from the pork source and not the refined and processed ones such as Crisco). Also since toxins oft times are stored in fat to protect the animal or person who is carrying it, we should make our animal fats come from trusted sources.

Most food companies and processors would have us think, it's best to drain off the fats, throw them away and replace with their oils that have healthy looking labels. These fats and oils have to be processed in a way to make them last longer, (hydrogenation of fats) which turns it into a fat that could be potentially harmful to your health!

Fat from its natural animal source, known as saturated fat, (pig fat, meat fats, dairy fats, fats in eggs etc.) are good for you, the problems mostly come in when we consume a lot of sugar and starches at the same time.

Most processed oils contain oxidized fats, (due to the refining process) and most all processed foods, as well as restaurant fryers use these oils as well. This can be pretty easy to avoid, by simply not eating fried foods from restaurants, avoiding processed foods, and avoiding using (most processed oils) in the home.

**Fat a vital nutrient:** fat is something that is very vital to health and we can rapidly lose our health, if we're not getting adequate amounts. It affects many functions such as regularity, building hormones, and is needed for cellular function in most of our, several trillion cells! The problem isn't fat from natural sources, its what the manufacturing processes do to the oils and fats to give it a longer shelf life that wind up causing problems in our arteries and veins.

**Good oils and fats to use or add:** butter - coconut oil - extra virgin olive oil (cold pressed) - avocado oil - non-hydrogenated lard - beef fat.

**Foods with good fats:** meats - eggs - dairy - nuts.

There are some oils we should simply avoid, especially if we have, or are trying to avoid heart related problems. The reason is because of the fats getting oxidized during the refining process and forming free radicals.

**Free radicals in fat:** the free radicals in oils developed under refining processes cause an inflammatory response throughout the body and when certain areas stay chronically inflamed for long enough (whether blood vessel, vital organs or skeletal system), it will lead to what later becomes diagnosed as a particular chronic disorder or disease. However, if you eat a lot of fruits, vegetables and other foods high in antioxidants, it may help you offset this.

**Bad oils:** instead of learning a long list of bad oils, I would rather point you in the direction of learning the above listed good fats and oils.

**How the good oils are made:** it's pretty neat that butter comes from cream that separates itself in milk naturally when raw milk sets for a while, and when the cream is shaken or stirred for a while turns into butter, olive and avocado oils can simply be cold pressed from its source instead of heat extraction. Coconut oil can be extracted by wet or dry processing.

By simply stocking our kitchen with the good oils, avoiding regular consumption of processed foods (almost all commercially processed foods have the bad fats in them) and eating less fried foods when we're away from home helps us eliminate a lot of the bad stuff.

Bottom line, the fats that naturally come with the foods we eat is a natural component of that food, making it a healthy source of fat. What makes it unhealthy is a high sugar and starch consumption with our fats!

# Gut Permeability and Autoimmune Diseases

When I was studying for my nutrition certification, the gastrointestinal tract and its processes impressed me more then anything in the entire course and has helped shape the way I look at food and the effects of nutrition.

Going step by step through the digestive processes was an amazing journey to me, and increased my faith that this powerful design came from Someone far greater then the result of a Big Bang or an evolving species.

The digestive part of our anatomy silently (or at least most times) processes the nutrients our body needs for building, re-building, energy and for fighting disease. The cool thing is how our body has its own system of checks and balances for our nutrient needs and will send orders to the digestive tract for the extraction and delivery of these nutrients, whenever it needs to build, energize or heal something in or on us.

The gastric system works the same as it did thousands of years ago, but there are some things that have changed in what our gut and intestinal tract recognizes as good food.

As Hippocrates said 2000 years ago... "All disease begins in the gut." This gives us a good reason to watch what goes into it, right?

**Irritable Bowel Syndrome (IBS):** is simply an immune reaction throughout our digestive tract and is caused most times by food and fluids that aggravate the lining of our gastrointestinal tract producing an inflammatory condition. And if we don't quit consuming the foods and fluids that cause this, it will become what we know as Irritable Bowel Syndrome (IBS). Keep in mind that inflammation in the digestive tract is no different then any other part of the body that gets inflamed in order to protect us from a source of aggravation. Just like any other part of the body, if it stays inflamed long enough (chronic inflammation) it can turn into a diseased body part, and our digestive tract is no different.

**Gluten and (IBS):** the reason gluten bothers some people's digestive tract, is because of it being a sticky protein, (gluten is a Latin term for glue). This gluten sticks to the walls of our digestive tract, causing some people great discomfort, (this is what we know as gluten intolerance). We would get really aggravated if we constantly got splattered with gluey goo, I would certainly get inflamed and probably just a little puffed up!

**Gut permeability:** imagine the area around a wound, how puffy and porous it gets, (this is simply inflammation going to work to help us in the healing process, after an acute injury). But when it happens continuously in the gut and our digestive tract stays puffy and porous, it allows food particles to enter the blood that have not been fully digested and OUR BLOOD IS SUPPOSED TO RECEIVE FOOD NUTRIENTS, NOT FOOD PARTICLES!!!

**Autoimmune disorders:** is something we should link directly to gut permeability. These food particles getting in the blood can be a contributing factor to disorders such as celiac disease, rheumatoid arthritis, type 1 diabetes, Hashimoto's thyroiditis, autoimmune cardiomyopathy, lymphoma, skin problems and more are caused primarily by systemic inflammatory conditions. Imagine how different parts of our body feel when they receive a food particle instead of broken down nutrients and oxygen like they're supposed to be getting. It probably makes the effected areas feel like our stomach does when it gets something it's not meant to digest.

**Sugar cravings:** when our gut becomes inflamed and leaky, it can also let yeast/candida into our bloodstream and since it feeds off of sugar, it can cause our cells to not get the glucose they should be getting to keep them energized.

**What you can do:** if you have an autoimmune disorder, switch over to a whole food diet and eliminate all processed foods from your diet. Using sprouted grain products can cut down on the gluten issue (the beginning stage of the sprouting process breaks down gluten, which makes it easier for us to digest). Keep a food diary, where you enter food, drink, the times you eat, and journal your water intake, (aim for a 1/2 oz. per pound of bodyweight). Write in how you feel upon waking, mid morning, noon, mid afternoon, early evening and at night, (this will show you the bad fuel that has been causing your engine to sputter).

We seriously need to stop eating and drinking the foods our digestive tract does not like, and just maybe we can quit taking medicines for the symptoms our gut is causing in other parts of the body! After all, it may taste good to the first 4 inches but how does it make the other 20 feet of our digestive tract feel?

Treating the symptoms of autoimmune disorders without changing our diet is like continuing to mop water up off the floor, while refusing to find and fix the leak.

# Greasy, Sugary Delicious Festival Food!

Fall brings in the cooler weather after a long hot summer as well as the beginning of the fall festivals and with these festivals comes the pizza, turkey legs, polish dogs, hot dogs, corn dogs fried candy bars, deep fried dill pickles, funnel cakes, kettle corn, caramelized and candied apples, many varieties of ice cream, (you can even get it fried), cobblers etc. These are only a few of the selections you have to choose from at the fair and it probably makes many of us get hungry just thinking about the food court area! If you've been to a festival here in the south, you probably know what it's like to be downwind from a Granny's Apple Dumplings!

If you read the above list of festival foods rapidly, it sounds like a massive train wreck of sugar and fat, right? I'm certainly not trying to advise anyone, not to eat the above, just a few hints on what you can do to keep from feeling like crud afterwards!

Have you ever noticed how you can eat something one day, and feel completely different eating the same thing on a different day? Very likely it's the energy deficit (lack of food) prior to eating, or energy expenditure (burning the food) after you ate it.

When we are really hungry (and not just because we smell good stuff cooking, baking or frying) but because we haven't eaten all day, our body will rapidly suck up the calories we consume. But if we eat several times prior to a calorie overload, we're apt to have horrible sugar spikes, (especially when consuming a lot of sugary foods) and if it's a lot of fat, its apt to sit like a brick in our stomach and an overall nasty feeling.

**These are a few things you can do:**

**1.** Skip eating at least one meal prior to event.

**2.** Exercise for 30-45 minutes using compound movements the day of event.

**3.** Plan to do a lot of walking at the event.

**4.** Space out the times and amounts you eat into smaller intervals.

**5.** You can also eat prior to going, (to cut food cravings) if you want to avoid these foods, or to eat controlled amounts at the festival.

**6.** If you are physically limited on exercise, walking etc., take some BeneFiber, Metamucil or other soluble fiber with you to the event. It is really easy to mix into your drink and is almost tasteless. This can really help control sugar spikes as well as having a cholesterol lowering effect. Bitter Mellon or cinnamon capsules can help control as well.

**7.** Last but not least and probably the most important, check the food vendor's setup for cleanliness and proper food rotation.

**After the binge:** whenever I've taken in way too many calories, I like to skip eating for a day, by doing an 18-24 hour intermittent fast.

# Breast Cancer Awareness Month

The month of October is selected for raising awareness and education in the fight against breast cancer, but the thing that really bothers me, is year by year it seems to be more and more about getting people into a detection and management cycle instead of prevention through education and lifestyle change.

**Questions:** the immune system is THE ONLY THING that heals the body, so when a person first gets diagnosed with cancer, why are they not immediately referred to a nutritionist who monitors blood work and nutritional intake for the next several months (after all, this helps fuel the immune system)? Since we know that sugar is cancer's primary fuel source, why don't we see if it shrinks or goes away without it? Should we not figure out what is causing the cancer first? Is cutting out a cancer, or trying to kill a cancer with radiation or chemotherapy drugs, not a little like smashing the light on a warning system, so we temporarily do not have to worry about what is going on behind the scenes? If you owned millions of dollars worth of diagnostic equipment, or were the patent owners of a multi-billion dollar drug or diagnostics machine, how would you want your advocates and lobbyists to indoctrinate?

**Example:** the sun and our body's natural production of vitamin D, has powerful anti-cancer effects in the body and is a powerful stimulant to our immune system, yet cancer industry groups such as the American Cancer Society run public service ads warning people about sunlight, but then do not warn people about the cancer causing chemicals in perfumes, laundry detergents and other personal care products, that may be sprayed or worn in and around breast tissue areas as well as other parts of the body.

A lot of the bend toward increasing awareness is simply to recruit more women into a cycle of repeat diagnostics and potentially as a customer in the form of radiation treatments, chemotherapy, or surgery with years of diagnostics and office visits to be scheduled after the poisonous and invasive procedures we have hook line and sinker, bought into.

Cancer and most chronic disease come from something that continues to cause aggravation either to an area or systemically in or on our body. Our body naturally forms a fibrin protein shield over an injured or aggravated area. If the aggravation continues, this shield will become tougher and harder to break down. If the inflammation that lies underneath continues to fester, due to the aggravation, it can slowly become a chronic condition that can eventually become a named cancer stemming from this area, whether breast, liver, lung etc.

Every one of us fights cancer everyday, the only time our body does not eradicate cancer is when our immune system is not strong enough for long enough, and if it cannot detect the cancer due to the fibrin protein shield it hides under. So should we not be learning and using these three primary things in our fight against cancer?

**1.** How do I stop aggravating this area or system of my body, so it will naturally shrink the cancer or tumor?

**2.** How do I build my immune system so it will stay strong enough for long enough?

**3.** How do I increase free circulating enzymes (Proteolytic) that will help strip away the fibrin shield the cancer hides and festers under so my immune system can attack it?

We know that most cancer builds itself from negative lifestyle habits, so could we not shrink and eradicate cancer by the opposite of that (positive lifestyle habits)?

# Health and Fitness...
# Trick or Treat?

There are some pretty serious tricks our body can start playing on us if we do not give it the simple things it wants from us, such as clean air, water, activity, rest, good diet, sunshine, deep sleep as well as stress relief and fun. When it comes to our body, we don't want it to reach into its dark and dismal bag of tricks, simply because we didn't give it the simple things it asks us for!

Many of us agree that when it's our time for our spirit to depart from this body, there is nothing going to stop it from happening, and though we have faith in much better things ahead but it still spooks most of us (at least a little) that we absolutely have no idea when or how this is going to happen. It's only human to want to live as long as possible.

Have you ever personally experience or watched someone else go through a health scare or crisis and suddenly things matter that didn't before and other things are no longer important. When health and mobility start failing, it does not matter who you are or what you have, things start aligning themselves.

Even if we continue to live despite our health failing us, we are simply living too short and dying too long.

The human anatomy is a mysterious one and is unmatchable in its capabilities both in physical performance and self-healing capabilities. But have you ever noticed how easy it is for someone to spook us about its weakness and incapability by using complicated words that name symptoms, diagnoses and then shrouding in mystery the things that are empowered by the simple and wholesome things (listed in the first paragraph). Our body has an immune system that turns the lights on throughout our innermost parts and is on guard 24-7-365 to protect us against the spoofers of good health!

**Health and fitness fear-mongering:** is used to produce a reaction and most times its done in a way to increase emotion along with speed of action, and not to increase a person's research, which is simply, lifestyle assessment and what is actually causing the problem.

When something scares us, we need to pull back from the situation, breath, relax and then research. Have you ever overreacted to something, which in turn caused a chain reaction of negative events? That's what can happen if we immediately run our body through all sorts of diagnostic machines and then start medicating with products that can have anywhere from 3-20 potential side effects.

**Masking:** a mask can make something that is good look bad, it can also cover up the bad with a mask that looks and feels good. This works much the same, when we medicate and manage symptoms without addressing what is causing the symptom.

**Example:** when we continue to take pain pills, we are simply masking the pain so we don't feel the inflammation and hurt our body or body part is going through. We should be babying our hurt body part along and start being extra nice to it, so it can heal; not going about life desensitized ourselves to this part of our body causing further damage. This keeps not only the pain going, but also increases inflammation, which is simply our body's healing response to injury. Pain has been given to us as a signal to STOP WHAT WE'RE DOING!

A healthy lifestyle is like a bag that holds the treats our body needs, (clean air, water, activity, balanced diet, sunshine, deep rest, stress relief and fun). These are the things that help keep it from playing tricks on us later!

# Fitness Recipes

Over the past 20+ years of being in the fitness business, I've come across about as many new ideas to train as diet fads that have come and gone. One of the main things I've learned is that one shoe doesn't fit all and a trainer should always listen to what his or her client's goals are and then design a program to get them there. This works the exact same way when a person wings it on his or her own whether in a gym or home exercise program.

The key to success in your fitness endeavors is figuring out exactly what you want from your fitness routine and then putting together a routine combined with a diet that will yield the results you want. It's a lot like a food recipe, if you don't use proper ingredients its not going to have the desired outcome.

Here are a few simple recipes for fitness, (I like using a little of each).

**Exercising to increase capabilities:** if someone wants to increase their physical capabilities in real life or in sports, they should do more compound (multiple joint) movements in their exercise routine and use free weights, (body weight exercises with increased speed of movement, and less rest time between sets help as well). Machines are great for toning and conditioning sections of the body, but they do very little for teaching muscle groups to contract and work together or to build stabilizer muscles like free weights do. Athletes and the elderly benefit a lot from the above style of exercising due to increased stability, core strength and muscles learning to work in a more powerful way together.

**For toning up:** when you do repeated sets stacked close behind each other for a particular body part it will cause this area to tone more rapidly.

**For strength:** increase the weight, this forces muscles to grow and accommodate. By increasing the workload, (whether in the amount of weight used or speed you move the weight) it increases power. This can be done with free weights, machines or bodyweight exercises. Keep in mind, machines do very little to strengthen stabilizer muscles (this is why an athlete can make a bodybuilder look clumsy).

**Bodybuilding:** to increase the size on a body part, you have to focus on pumping that muscle or muscle group up. The pump, the intense straining, muscle breakdown causes the body to build itself back stronger to accommodate the new workload. Muscle does NOT care how it looks, just that it is able to accommodate increased workloads. Carb loading prior to workouts and an increased intake of protein and fats are important for fuel, muscle repair and for building hormones.

**Burning body fat:** exercising more rapidly is the way to go if you want to trigger the fat burn state. Fat release for energy happens around 20 minutes into your exercise routine, (this is what is happening when we feel our 2nd wind kick in).

**Cardiovascular endurance:** exercise with lighter weights, compound movements and exercise faster with less rest between sets. I have for a long time tried to get members to blur the lines between the cardio room, and the rest of the gym. In other words, if you want to build muscle and strength, lift weights, if you want to build cardio strength, lift weights faster and with less rest! Exercising faster with less rest between sets using compound movements does 4 things at one time, increases strength, muscle size, cardiovascular endurance and burns fat. This is much more applicable to real life then jogging for 5-10 miles.

**Final recipe:** Exercising and stretching from the different angles you use in real life (combined with a good diet, recovery and deep sleep), will yield strength, increased physical capabilities that enhance your life, increased muscle and bone density, flexibility, improved lean weight to body fat ratio, slow the aging process, increased metabolism, decreased stress levels as well as many other physiological benefits!!!

# Cold Weather Increases Thermogenesis

A cold November wind blew in on the 1st, like it had been waiting for the date to change! Fall is my favorite time of year, but not so much for others, including a friend and member that assured me the other morning that I can expect her to be complaining until spring! However there is a bright side to a long winter for anyone that wants to shed body fat before coming out of hibernation next spring and summer!

**Cold weather thermogenesis:** thermogenesis is a process when the body generates heat and it does this by burning calories, which are units of heat.

When your body is exposed to cold, it burns calories (like heating fuel) to keep your body warmed to the temperature it's supposed to stay at (around 98.6°). Calories are units of heat and since we burn more of them during the wintertime when we have increased cold exposure, we are apt to see an increase in our appetite. If we drop our caloric intake every so often, our body will look elsewhere for calories.

**Borrowing calories from fat:** this is how we decrease our fat storage and if we temporarily cut our calories down (especially calories from sugar) our body will make up for this deficit by releasing calories from our fat cells, thus deflating them.

External cold temperatures has a lot the same calorie burning effect as drinking cold water, either way our body has to try to maintain a body temperature of around 98.6° and whatever lowers this temperature will trigger thermogenesis. Water has been shown to increase the metabolic rate by 30% after drinking 500 ml (little over 2 cups) during a 40-minute period. 40% of this increase comes from warming the water.

**Our thermostat:** we have a really cool thermostat in our brain called the hypothalamus and it is responsible for regulating temperature control among many other things throughout the body. So the next time you start shivering, you will know your thermostat has turned on the heat and the fuel used is calories (whether it comes from your digestive tract or stored calories from fat).

**Night time temperatures:** a recent study showed an increase in burning body fat throughout the night in both men and women, by dropping temperature from 75° to 67°.

Just like our fireplace will use up the wood we have stock piled to keep our house warm during the winter, we can also manipulate our calorie intake so that our body will burn stored fat to keep us warm.

We can use the cold weather to enhance our weight loss goals, so when we come out of hibernation in March we'll be ready for spring and summer!!! Or not, (there's always the alternative of building up some good thick natural thermal wear underneath our skin).

# Heart Warming Effects of
# The Cayenne Pepper

Cayenne pepper is not only great for spicing up food, the stack of health benefits seem to be as high as the heat in this pepper! The list of health benefits and remedies is a long one but the powerful cardiopulmonary effects of this pepper really stood out to me.

Heart disease is the number 1 leading killer of Americans, (the way things are now, 1 of 3 of us will die from it) so a recent article title caught my attention "Cayenne Pepper - Stop a heart attack fast." The next paragraph is a clip from someone that was famous for healing and teaching, and the name doctor was one that was earned only, (not licensed by today's standards of medical practice).

Dr. John Christopher a famed healer and American Herbalist (1909-1983) said: "In 35 years of practice, and working with the people and teaching, I have never on house calls lost one heart attack patient, and the reason is, whenever I go -if they are still breathing -I pour down them a cup of cayenne tea (a teaspoon of cayenne in a cup of hot water, and within minutes they are up and around).

Have you ever drunk a warm cup of water and cayenne pepper? I did and I can certainly understand why they were up and around within minutes!

I do not know why it seems to have such a powerful effect on stopping or potentially preventing heart attack, but there are a few factual elements I stitched together that seem to really add logic to this.

**Key effects:** cayenne pepper rapidly equalizes blood pressure in the arterial and venous system - it warms the body - dilates blood vessels - is a general nervous stimulant - helps with muscle cramps - increases circulation and blood flow to all major organs which facilitates oxygen and nutrient delivery. When the heart stops functioning, our capability to deliver oxygen and nutrients to all parts of the body cease and without oxygen and nutrients we die rapidly!

Some nutrients are quite powerful in how they affect certain functions of the body. Some of the primary ones in cayenne pepper are **vitamin A, vitamin B6, vitamin C, riboflavin, potassium,** and **manganese**. I wanted to find out what effect these main nutrients in cayenne pepper had on the heart, so I researched them individually.

This is what I found;

**Vitamin A:** good for protecting the heart and cardiovascular system.

**Vitamin B6:** vitamin B6 (Pyridoxine) used for heart disease, high cholesterol, reducing blood levels of homocysteine (a chemical that might be linked to heart disease) and helping clogged arteries stay open after a balloon procedure to unblock them (angioplasty).

**Vitamin C:** is used for hardening of the arteries, preventing clots in veins and arteries, heart attack, stroke, high blood pressure, and high cholesterol.

**Riboflavin:** used for muscle cramps, required for proper development of blood cells, and increases red blood cell's ability to release oxygen to tissues of the body.

**Potassium:** used to treat high blood pressure and prevent stroke.

**Manganese:** used for tired blood (anemia), PMS and is an essential nutrient for processing cholesterol.

I really thought it was awesome that, as I broke down and researched the individual nutrient elements to see why the cayenne pepper is so effective for the heart, a multi-vitamin for the heart seemed came together in front of my own eyes! Cayenne pepper definitely seems to be nature's nitroglycerine, so if you worry about a potential heart attack, keep some cayenne (and some water to mix it with) close!

The list of health benefits of cayenne pepper is an extensive one and much too long to include here, but it truly is a medicinal gift from nature!

Cayenne pepper (capsicum) may very well be nature's multi-vitamin for the heart, but this is just one example of the powerful medicinal effect that foods can have on the body, in both prevention and healing!

**Note:** cayenne pepper is also available in capsule form.

**Warning:** do not drink coffee right after taking cayenne capsules, it doesn't feel good at all!

# Holiday Food Hangovers

I'm sure many of us are looking forward to a BIG Thanksgiving feast (or several) and some good family time, but how many of us feel like sleeping instead of visiting once we get through eating?

We often hear it blamed on the tryptophan in the turkey and how it induces sleepiness, but it's a whole lot more about how much we ate. Turkey actually has less tryptophan in it then chicken does, and we don't often hear someone blaming chicken for making him or her sleepy.

When we eat a lot of heavy foods, two things usually happen;

**1.** Spikes in our blood sugar levels and then the subsequent crashes.

**2.** A diversion of energy going to our digestive tract.

**Sugar spikes:** when we have a lot of sugar or foods that are breaking down into sugar, our body pours insulin into our bloodstream to transport the sugars, and this insulin will continue to look for sugar in the blood until it is convinced that there is no more sugar left to transport. This is what causes the crash.

**Diversion of energy:** we burn a lot of energy when we digest food, this is especially so when we eat a lot of heavy food and gives some really good logic to the siesta (after lunch nap). Imagine your gut being a distribution warehouse and everything else being a complex network of highways and railways to transport nutrients to their respective destinations and the liver, kidneys, and lymphatic system being a state of the art waste processing and elimination system. The digestive and elimination processes take a lot of energy and this energy demand grows in lock step with the amount and types of food we eat.

Most of us want to loosen up on our diet around the holidays, but dread the stuffed, tired feeling, here are a few simple things we can do to avoid this, and still eat as much as we want to.

## Avoiding a food hangover:

**1.** Avoid sugar when eating a high fat and high starch meal.

**2.** Skip a meal before the big one and the one after.

**3.** Increase activity before the meal and within 60-90 minutes after the meal, (this is when blood sugar peaks).

**4.** Soluble fiber such as BeneFiber or Metamucil helps coat food and slows down absorption, (mixing and drinking some with a meal slows down the sugars and has a cholesterol lowering effect with high fat meals).

**5.** Eat some raw vegetables along with the heavy stuff, (it helps move big sticky globs along through the digestive tract).

Doing some intense activity just before a meal activates GLUT4 receptors, which helps our body, suck up energy into muscle throughout our body and lowers the need for so much insulin production from our pancreas. This also helps us avoid pumping up our fat cells with a lot of extra calories from our food.

Note: doing these things also can help a diabetic person lower their need for insulin.

**Example exercises:** anything that can get a lot of muscles working like bodyweight squats, air jumps, pushups and jumping jacks, or a full body workout using resistance training, will fire up these GLUT4 receptors, burn off extra calories and will help you feel so much better. Doing the above will definitely jump start your calorie furnace!

# Chicken Soup for the Immune System

When our immune system is fending off or defending us from invaders, it needs energy and its energy need increases in direct proportion to the battle it is fighting!

Have you ever noticed how your energy for your regular external activities goes down, for no apparent reason? This can happen if you unknowingly made contact with and are fighting a virus, bacterial infection or such things as cancer cell growth. Our body and its immune system are really good at multi-tasking, but sometimes it would probably like to be able to say, I can't right now...we're busy!

Our digestive tract consumes a lot of energy to break down and digest the nutrients out of the foods we eat and then to process and eliminate the waste. If we can lighten this load, more of our energy can go to our immune system.

There was research published in the American Journal of Therapeutics that documented that a compound in chicken soup called carnosine can help strengthen the body's immune system to fight off flu in the early stages. But for this to work, you'll need to consume a steady supply throughout your illness for the effect to work, is the authors claim. Chicken has about 2,000 mg per pound, however I personally believe the effects of the other components in the chicken, and the other supplemental ingredients in the chicken soup, makes the carnosine more effective when gotten through food then in the supplement form of carnosine.

**The recipe that was used in the study:**
chicken, onions, parsnips, turnips, carrots, celery, stems, parsley, salt and pepper, but a similar effect was found from canned soup.

I like the above recipe, because it gets a lot of nutrients combined that should boost the body's nutrient levels in the blood and since the ingredients are softened, it should be very easy on the digestive tract which in turn means you can direct more energy to what your immune system is fighting.

Two of the main things our immune system needs from us when it is working on a tough internal battle, is rest and good nutrition that is easy to process. We need to choose foods that are low in refined sugar and carbs, but high in nutrition.

**According to a study by Loma Linda University,** sugar has been shown to slow down the activity of our white blood cells (our immune system's defenders). So eliminating any refined sugar is key, especially if you want your immune system to rise to win its battles. Dumping sugar into our system depresses the immune system by about 30% and consistent sugar consumption keeps it permanently depressed. The intestinal tract is a major part of our immune system and needs healthy gut flora to stimulate the production of immune cells and plays a major role in digesting and eliminating the bad stuff (carcinogens) in our diet. A high sugar diet kills off this intestinal flora and when this happens it compromises our immune system and lets pathogens such a yeast (candida) to grow!

**If you take an antibiotic:** it is important after oral antibiotic usage, to get a good source of probiotics (supplements, probiotic rich foods such as fermented vegetables, yogurt etc.) to undo the digestive tract damage the antibiotics have done.

If you keep the body strong enough for long enough, the immune system will learn and then outsmart the invader (things that cause sickness and disease) with the perfect medicine (antibodies etc.) designed by your body's own personal pharmacy!

# Limited Medical Access May Cure More People

I do not want to offend anyone; this article is only to provoke thought and possibly some action...

Just recently I read an article about a stance that is being taken against a new wave of expensive drugs, some as high as $50,000 a month! This is a form of life support that is probably not going to be sustainable and with the new structure of government subsidized healthcare will transfer a massive amount of wealth to pharmaceutical companies and their shareholders at the expense of the taxpayers in this country.

If we do not embrace prevention, personal responsibility and cures instead of (early detection and its ensuing counterpart of managing chronic conditions and disease), we are going to have a diseased fiscal problem in this country, as well as continued growth of current and new chronic diseases. We will very likely see employers running their companies just to pay the pharmacy bill, and many small to medium size businesses will probably be wiped out, (the money has to come from somewhere)!

Continuing to develop drugs and expensive diagnostic procedures for a society of people unwilling to help themselves has grown into something that is probably not going to be sustainable.

Pharmaceutical companies have developed drugs that can help us deal with almost any lifestyle choices we have made and want to continue. This has caused many of us to adapt a mentality, that even if we're not good stewards of our health, the medical system will fix and then maintain us.

**Example:** Nexium tops the pharmaceutical list at $5.276 Billion in sales. Nexium helps people deal with excessive stomach acid, which is probably directly linked to, processed low enzyme foods, loads of sugar and a fast food diet guzzled down with acidic, carbonated, caffeinated, sugar loaded sodas. Lipitor is next at $5.272 Billion in sales. Lipitor is a statin designed to lower blood fats, which is directly linked to diet as well. OxyContin has the number 5 slot on the list at $3.554 Billion in sales, and is only one out of the many legal addictive pharmaceutical narcotic pain drugs. Pretty easy to see why it's illegal to grow your own for free.

One industry that is literally exploding in sales and profits is the one for treating and managing cancer. This is a huge market since everyone that is alive fights cancer, so if you're alive, you are a potential customer. This has grown from 5 cancer drugs in the 70's at a median monthly cost of $129 per month for treatment to 33 cancer drugs in 2014 and $9,905 per month. This is over a 900,000% increase in costs. With all this money spent, why is death from cancer on the rise? According to the CDC one out of every four deaths in the United States is from cancer. Should we not be looking for what is causing cancer, instead of a cure for cancer?

Shouldn't we look for ways to poison our body less instead of more?

Treating symptoms is like being given a bucket to deal with a leaking pipe, instead of using the right tools and material to fix the pipe. When we are told that we cannot get expensive medicine for something, it will force us to think about what we can do to lower our need for it.

**Example:** when you are told you're borderline diabetic, this most likely is coming from a body growing weary of all the sugars and starches in your diet with very little fiber to slow down the sugar after consumption. A lot of people qualify for drugs such as metformin and other anti diabetic drugs, and a lot of people would rather take these drugs then change what they eat. Many of these drugs simply lower your sugar in your blood to safe levels but are not designed to cure the problem.

**Example:** if you sprain your ankle, what does it need from you to help it feel better? Does it want a drug in your system to desensitize you to the pain it is feeling? Or would your ankle rather you lighten up the load on it and put a support around it to hold it immobile while it is trying to recover? Masking the pain with a pain pill would probably let you continue putting pressure on this area, further injuring it, but then that makes you a better continuing customer for the pain management industry right?

When we are told that we can no longer get a medicine, or told a certain procedure will not be available for us, it helps us become proactive in doing things that go to the root of the problem. This eliminates the symptoms and DRIES OUT THE PROBLEM!!! This can be for something as simple as wearing a support belt for a hurting back or keeping a food log to figure out what foods or fluids are giving us digestive issues.

Are you on a drug that gives your life support? Are you guaranteed a life supply of this drug that you are growing dependence on? Is there a lifestyle change you can make that will decrease your dependence on this drug? Isn't continuing to treat symptoms a little like unplugging the check engine light that keeps coming on?

# Muscle Does Not Care
# How It Looks...

 Muscle does not care how it looks, only that it can handle the workload better. Muscle tone and the size increase is simply muscle adapting to what you regularly make it do. If we never challenge our muscle(s) its conditioning will not improve and if we do not at least keep them active with our own bodyweight, even our own body will begin to feel heavy to itself.

 Have you ever noticed the difference in a bodybuilder and a long distance runner? The bodybuilder's muscles have gotten big to accommodate the heavy workload and the long distance runner becomes very lean, with much smaller muscles that are efficient for going a long time and distance.

Even if we're doing it for the tone, the shape, or the size, our muscle cares nothing about the above three, only that it is able to better handle the workload we put on it.

Without the bones, our body would be a big puddle of muscle, skin and organs, but without muscle our bones would be unable to move, so it takes these two working together (with the stimulus of nerves) to help us carry out our activities.

**Activities of daily living (ADL's):** when our muscles regularly contract doing the daily things we deem necessary, our muscles stay toned to maintain this level of demand, but if we discontinue, these things become harder whenever we decide we want to do them again, (this applies to most anything, including sports).

If you want to build your physical capabilities to (more easily) carry out your daily routine, you can either intensify your daily activities or add in an exercise program that works your muscles in much the same way as you expect to use them in real life.

**Preconditioning:** preconditioning works really well if you know there is an event coming up that will be physically taxing. Simply doing things that mimic the future stress and then doing them with consistency trains and conditions your mind and body. This helps prevent excessive tiredness, acute injury, and chronic inflammatory joint problems and you can enjoy the event much more as well because you've preconditioned your muscles to handle it better.

**Example:** if you have a trail hike coming up with a group of friends, the best way to train for that is walking around your yard, up and down hills and other uneven surfaces NOT a track or a treadmill.

**Example:** if you have a sedentary job, and you're going to have to move to another house, start lifting and carrying heavier things in the preceding weeks to condition yourself for the unusually stressful day coming up.

When we start making our body work harder in our exercise conditioning program, over time we will not only notice the activity getting easier, we'll also see the muscles we're using for this activity, tone and build as well!

Muscle does not care what it looks like, only that it is able to handle the job better, so if you want it to change its shape, force it to do work that it is not used to!

# A Year in Review...Fit-Notes for the New Year

This article is simply a recap of some of this past year's articles, and I'll try to keep it as condensed as possible and for most that know me know that is a little hard for me to do...

**1.** Our body craves: clean air, water, balanced diet, sunshine, activity, rest and less stress. The basics still work, are not expensive and are the best medicine.

**2.** Fat and mucous helps shield us from toxins: detoxing helps with weight loss and helps keep these toxins from aging us while we're shedding fat. Eat plenty of fiber while detoxing and losing weight, or the toxins will reabsorb into your system. Fiber helps drag toxins out through your waste.

**3.** Sugar makes you fatter then fat: your body has to pull excess sugar from your blood that you're not burning and it will store the extra in your fat cells.

**4.** Your body is made up with a completely new generation of cells every year: your lifestyle habits pretty much dictate their revitalization or deterioration.

**5.** When trying to find out which exercise program is best for you, look to your lifestyle specific needs: when we know exactly what we are wanting, (whether it's weight loss, strengthening, building, cardiopulmonary conditioning or a combination of either of the above), all we have to do is add in the program that works best for us and fits into our life. We are not designed to fit in someone else's shoe.

**6.** A shrinking of muscle decreases physical capabilities, increased muscle and tone increases capability: regular activity tones and conditions the muscles to continue handling this level of stress.

**7.** We have free fat burners available: 1. Temporary calorie restriction causes your body to release calories from fat cells, 2. Our body burns calories to keep us warm. 3. Our body burns a lot of calories when we eat foods that break down slower vs. foods that turn to a starchy or sugary mush as soon as we eat them.

**8.** Instead of treating inflammation, how bout we get rid of the aggravation that is causing the inflammation. Inflammation is actually a part of the healing process, but if not turned off, will continue festering until it turns into a diseased condition. Get rid of the aggravation, you then get rid of the inflammation which dries out the chronic diseased condition.

**9.** Antidepressants are known to give people suicidal thoughts: have you tried healthy diet and exercise?

**10.** Supplements are gap fillers: knowing what gaps you're trying to fill can save you money and keep your body from having to detox itself from things it doesn't need.

**11.** Instability in exercise (free weights, bodyweight exercises, etc.) helps us with greater stability in real life. Machines do not do much in strengthening our stabilizer muscles.

**12.** Pushups, squats and planks are some of the best exercises you can do at home. Your body is your universal gym. Note: we should practice getting up from the floor more often; it exercises most of your body's muscles when you do this.

**13.** Heart Disease and Cancer are the leading killers: the leading cause of heart disease and cancer is lifestyle.

**14.** Green leafy vegetables help gives us clearer vision: they contain large amounts of the eye's favorite antioxidants, (lutein and zeaxanthin).

**15.** There is a bonus payout on jobs that require manual labor: you get to exercise on the job and probably have better health then the average person that sits behind a desk, (especially ones who do not exercise).

**16.** Pain pills are blinders of fact: they desensitize us to a body part that is screaming out in pain. It's like putting earmuffs on when your child is screaming and acting like everything is okay because you can't hear anything. Wrap it, support it, massage it, cool it, being nice to it your hurting body part helps heal it.

**17.** If health seems to be getting off track: start a food, hydration, activity and sleep journal.

**18.** Buy produce as much as you can from people you know: when they grow foods for their own consumption, you can trust it much more then produce that comes through food market logistics.

**19.** Up and down movement is what stimulates the flow of lymph fluid in our lymphatic system: this is a big part of our waste removal system and much of our immune system. Jumping jacks, trampoline, most free weight and bodyweight exercises that cause intense muscle contractions, will help move lymph fluid upwards as well.

**20.** All disease begins in the gut: if we have digestive problems, we should get to the bottom of it as soon as possible. Antibiotics are anti-gut health; probiotic rich foods are pro gut health. If you need to take antibiotics, eat probiotic rich foods and take a probiotic supplement to restore gut and digestive health.

**21.** We should research for what's causing things instead of trying to cure them.

**22.** When your body is fighting the flu, lighten up on the foods you eat (soups, jello, broths etc.) this will let more energy go to your immune system, instead of digestion.

**23.** Less medicine and medical access would make us more proactive in adopting healthy preventive lifestyle habits

**24.** Muscle does not care what it looks like: it only cares that it is able to better handle the stress we regularly put it through.

# The Power In Strong Muscle And Strong Blood!

Healthier, stronger, faster, leaner, and more muscular with stronger connective tissue, is what many of us have as part of our resolutions for the New Year. These are very good ones to make, since they help us to stay physiologically younger, in better shape, help us avoid injury, make us more capable, and help our body's immune system fight chronic disease, instead of managing it with medical care.

A resolution is much like a recipe, it's made up of ingredients that create the end product. Once we have the ingredients together, we have to put it into action, by using required amounts, mixing them for consistency and then baking or cooking it, without overdoing it! Your fitness goals are no different, and even though we oft times remake the same fitness goals of the prior year; they're well worth remaking.

We may not have reached our actual goals, but we may have slowed things up a bit or maybe even headed it in the right direction. We might know what we didn't accomplish, but we don't usually get to see what we prevented.

**Finding your health and fitness recipe:** most of us know what we have to do, unless we have a chronic or complicated condition and even then, most times the basic ingredients for health and fitness apply. For most of us, simply cleaning up our intake and increasing our activity yields great results when done with consistency. If you need a coach for the above, a good trainer and someone certified or knowledgeable in nutrition can help you put together an action plan. Just remember, the basic fundamentals are easy and they work better then complicated routines, and complicated nutrition plans. Confusion is meant to benefit the one selling you the goods and services not you...

**Exercise action plan:** I would like to see each of us be able to do more of at least 3 things at the end of each year; more squats, more pushups, and a longer duration of doing the plank. As we become stronger, I would like to see us all able to do the pushups and squats faster or with greater resistance, such as free weight bench press and barbell squats. Remember that doing your bodyweight faster creates greater resistance also, so you do not have to have exercise equipment or gym access for any of the above. You can also turn manual work around the house and on the job into an exercise routine as well by increasing your speed and workload. Gradually increase resistance and speed of movement to avoid injury. Small increases when done consistently, really adds up over the course of a year. This action plan will help strengthen muscles, bones and connective tissue. It also increases blood circulation to body parts starving for nutrients and oxygen, thus lowering the risk of disease in these areas.

**Nutrition action plan:** keeping a good variety of foods in your diet is key to good health and your body's capability to fight disease. Eat less processed foods and try to eat more locally grown ones. Food that does well in an area help us do well. If you do not have a garden, find someone that does and arrange to purchase from them. Purchasing from them is better then getting it from them for free, this makes it worth their time to plant or grow more the next year.

Remember, there is a nutrition plan for almost every fitness goal, chronic condition, or disease. Hippocrates said let thy food be thy medicine and thy medicine be thy food, this applies to supplements as well. There is value in both, but we should remember first and foremost that there is power in food and making nutrition a part of our action plan will help build strong blood and a strong immune system, and this can help your body fight disease better then any pharmacy on earth!

**Stress action plan:** mental stress is probably one of the biggest indirect killers among us. It is also a major cause in retaining fat in the abdominal area. Mental stress needs to be combined with physical exertion in order to keep it from building up inside us, causing hormonal imbalances and toxic side effects. Keeping stress levels low should be a part of any health and fitness routine, it helps with lowering our body fat, and lowers our risk of chronic disease.

Lets try to breathe more clean air, drink clean fluids (water), eat more locally grown foods, become stronger, healthier, get out in the sun more, get deeper sleep, stress less and subsequently spend less time in doctor's offices (on chronic disease witch hunts) and the ensuing chronic disease managed care.

When you keep your body healthy and strong, it not only helps maintain good shape, it also unleashes its capabilities to fight premature aging and disease!

Our body is designed to be a survival machine with an Internal Doctor that works 24-7-365 so whatever our starting point is, lets give it the tools it needs to do its job!!!

I wish you all the best in health & Fitness! Wade Yoder

## About the author

Wade Yoder has been in the health and fitness club business since 1991 and is a weekly health and fitness columnist for 5 Middle, Georgia newspapers with over 160 published articles since 2012.
He owns and operates Valley Athletic Club in Fort Valley, Georgia